The
One-Minute[*]
Cleaner
Plain & Simple

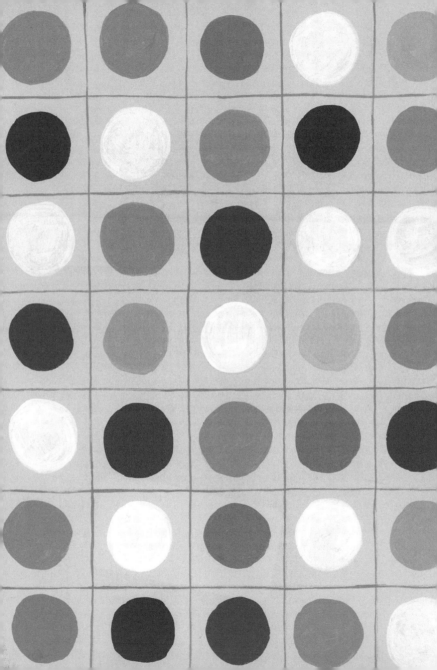

The One-Minute Cleaner

Plain & Simple

BY DONNA SMALLIN

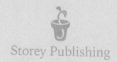

Storey Publishing

*The mission of Storey Publishing is to serve our customers by
publishing practical information that encourages
personal independence in harmony with the environment.*

Edited by Nancy D. Wood and Rebekah Boyd-Owens
Cover design and art direction by Vicky Vaughn
Cover and interior illustrations © 2006 by Juliette Borda
Text production by Jennifer Jepson Smith, based on design
  by Wendy Palitz
Indexed by Mary McClintock

Printed in the United States by Versa Press
10 9 8 7 6 5 4 3 2 1

Library of Congress Cataloging-in-Publication Data

Smallin, Donna, 1960–
    The one-minute cleaner : plain and simple / by Donna Smallin.
        p. cm.
    Includes bibliographical references and index.
    ISBN-13: 978-1-58017-659-0; ISBN-10: 1-58017-659-3 (pbk. : alk. paper)
    1. House cleaning I. Title.
TX324.S535 2007
648'.5—dc22
                                                            2007000334

contents

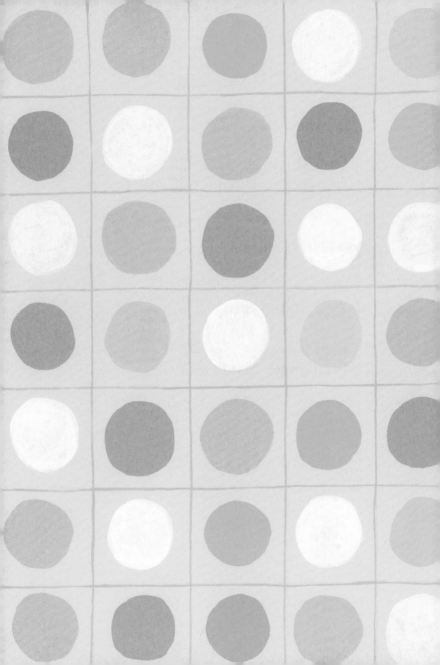

Into every life a little dirt will fall. Add a layer of dust, a few stains, a dash of greasy grime, and now you have a real job on your hands. The problem is you also have a busy lifestyle, which doesn't leave much time or energy to deal with everyday grunge. You end up spending a good deal of your free time cleaning (or feeling guilty that you aren't clean- ing). Or you attempt to keep up as best you can, hoping all the while that you will someday have time to catch up.

Housekeeping is one of those jobs that's never done. In fact, in many homes it's a job that's barely begun. Working women have all but aban- doned their traditional role of head housekeeper. Spouses and children have taken up some of the workload, but still, not everything that should be done is getting done. By choice or necessity, standards have been relaxed to accommodate busy schedules that frequently force domestic responsibilities to the bottom of the to-do list.

The simplest solution to the cleaning quandary is to learn how to get your housecleaning done faster, so you can spend more of your free time doing what you'd rather be doing! That's the purpose of this book — to provide plain and simple cleaning practices, techniques, and strategies that make quick work of housework.

A Clean House, One Small Task at a Time

The One-Minute Cleaner Plain & Simple is written for busy people who want a clean home *and* a life. You'll find hundreds of practical tips and ideas for cleaning everything from kitchen counters to eyeglass lenses, from outdoor decks to bird cages. And because it takes individual lifestyles and special needs into consideration, this book also includes cleaning tips for allergy sufferers, strategies to ensure the safety of children in the home, and natural nontoxic "green" cleaning recipes.

I've always found cleaning to be therapeutic for the body, mind, and soul. I believe many of us are striving to cope with a chaotic world. We may not be able to stop war or terrorism, and we certainly can't keep hurricanes and earthquakes from occurring, but we can clean up our own little corner of the world.

This book is divided into two parts: Ready, Set, Clean! and Challenges Inside and Out. Chapters include strategies for getting on top of the house-work load and ongoing maintenance for every living space you occupy. Most pages offer practical advice for any day of the week, any time of the day, and a few are geared toward seasonal cleaning or preparing for special occasions. Every tip can be read in seconds; many implemented in as little as one minute. Look for the one-minute symbol ☀①.

Whatever your cleaning goals, know that the only standards that matter are those you set for yourself. Whether you enjoy cleaning or do anything you can to avoid it, there's no point in making it any harder than it has to be. Armed with proven tips, techniques, and strategies, you'll be able to accomplish every cleaning task in record time and with less effort than you ever imagined possible.

PART ONE

Ready, Set, Clean!

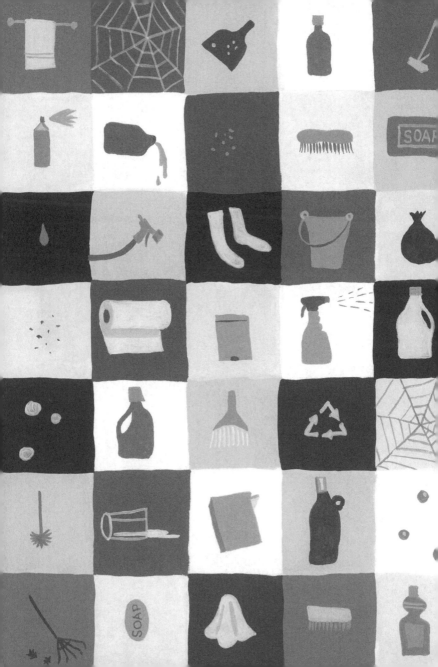

CHAPTER 1

Make a Plan

You don't need a degree in housekeeping to maintain a clean, uncluttered home. You also don't need to spend all your spare time cleaning. What you do need are the right tools and supplies, an understanding of how to best use them, and a plan for what you hope to accomplish. Most people would probably enjoy living in a clean home — if only they didn't have to work! Guess what? It might not be as hard as you think.

Ask yourself why you clean? What's in it for you? Would you like to be able to eat off the floors? Or would you be happy just to be able to fix dinner without having to clean up the kitchen or empty a sink full of dishes first?

What are **your goals** for cleaning?

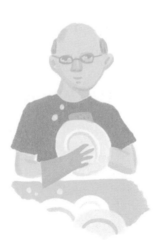

make a plan

What are the benefits to cleaning? First and foremost, a clean home is a **healthier home.** Germs in your home can create and spread illness. While it is impossible to kill all germs, cleaning and disinfecting is the best offense against them.

☀ ❶ Cleaning is an **investment.** Regular upkeep helps carpets and furnishings last longer. Frequent vacuuming can extend the life of carpets by preventing dirt from being ground in, which can destroy carpet fibers, for example. A regular cleaning routine can save you money in the long run.

make a plan

Know, exactly, what you are cleaning:

- **Dirt** comes into the house on our shoes, clothes, and hair. It consists of accumulated crumbs, pet hair, pest droppings, and other undesirable matter we can wipe, sweep, or vacuum up.

- **Dust** is a combination of many things, including feather and fabric fibers, pet dander, food particles, insect parts, and microscopic mites.

- **Germs** are potentially harmful microorganisms, including bacteria and viruses, that cause illnesses that can be transmitted via unclean surfaces.

- **Mold,** like germs, is a natural part of our environment, but it can cause allergic responses and asthma attacks.

**The look and smell
of a freshly cleaned
home produces a sense
of accomplishment,
SATISFACTION,
and pride.**

make a plan

Our cleaning approach depends on our attitudes, **preferences,** experience, time, energy, and goals. Most of us fall into one of four categories: speed cleaner, green cleaner, super cleaner, or catch-up cleaner.

Speed cleaners who desire a clean house, but place cleaning activities low on their priority list, should start with a thorough cleaning and then get into the habit of doing a little each day.

❶ Speed cleaners might use a caddy to tote supplies and products like disinfectant wipes for quick cleanups.

Many commercial products contain natural ingredients, but **green cleaners** looking for a cleaning approach that is kinder to the earth will find items in their kitchen cabinets that do the job just as well. For example, white vinegar and water can be used to clean counters and floors. And baking soda is the perfect nonabrasive cleaner for the kitchen and bath.

MAKE YOUR OWN
All-Purpose Green Cleaner

❶ Combine 1 teaspoon of vegetable oil-based laundry detergent, 1 teaspoon of borax laundry detergent, and 2 tablespoons of white vinegar with 1 quart of hot water.

Go easy with damaging products if you're a **super cleaner** who tends to clean with a vengeance. Start each project with the least harsh cleaning solution. Be sure to disinfect oft-used kitchen sponges and towels (see page 78) or you will spread more germs while you work.

❶ If cleaning starts to feel like an obsession, recognize that you may be using it as an excuse to avoid dealing with something else.

make a plan

Catch-up cleaners who have a fairly high tolerance for dirt, dust, and clutter might consider hiring help or arrange a work trade with family members or friends to get the house clean. Then clean a little bit every day.

Set a timer for 10 minutes in the morning and 10 minutes at night and clean, clean, clean. Use the first 10 minutes to clean your bathroom or kitchen and the second 10 for a bigger chore, such as vacuuming.

Offer yourself a daily reward for your efforts.

It's a lot easier to

KEEP UP than

to catch up.

make a plan

While cleaning with soap and water will *remove* most germs from surfaces, disinfectants effectively *kill* germs. It's a good idea to always disinfect surfaces in the kitchen, bathroom, and nursery.

To properly **disinfect** surfaces, clean and wash them with a cleaning solution to remove soils, and then spray or wipe it with a diluted bleach solution or a ready-made disinfectant. Let the surface air-dry or wipe it dry with a clean cloth or paper towel.

1 If a household member is sick, you can **reduce the risk** of spreading viruses and bacteria by disinfecting frequently touched surfaces such as light switches, doorknobs, remote controls, and telephone receivers.

A commonly used disinfectant is liquid chlorine bleach, but be aware that bleach only has a 3- to 6-week shelf life, and consider that the bottle spent time on a shelf before you bought it.

make a plan

Spend a little time each day cleaning. Modify the following everyday to-do list to suit your needs and lifestyle:

- Make all the beds.
- Empty wastebaskets as needed.
- Round up dirty laundry.
- Wipe bathroom sinks.
- Sweep the kitchen floor.
- Vacuum carpets in high-traffic areas as needed.
- Clean the kitchen table and countertops.
- Wash dishes.
- Start a wash, load and start the dryer, or fold laundry as needed.
- Sort mail into categories: to pay, to file, to read, to call, or to trash or recycle.
- Pick up clutter.

Make It Easier

☀ **Challenge** yourself to make your bed in less than 60 seconds.

☀ Wipe bathroom sinks in the morning before leaving the room.

Clean up the kitchen after dinner.

Carry a trash bag from room to room and empty all the wastebaskets. Pick up clutter before heading to bed. Get the idea?

You need to develop and implement a **cleaning plan** for those chores that require time and effort on a regular basis, such as mopping floors or cleaning your refrigerator. Most homes can be maintained with once-a-week cleaning. However, how often you tackle regular cleaning chores largely depends on how many people are living in your home. If you have children or pets, you probably need to vacuum and mop more than once a week. If you live alone without pets, you might be able to squeak by on a biweekly cleaning schedule provided you pick up clutter every day.

Following are three ways to approach weekly cleaning chores:

Plan 1: All at Once.
This traditional approach to weekly cleaning works well for people who have two or more days off each week and either enjoy cleaning or enjoy the satisfaction that comes from cleaning the whole house from top to bottom.

Plan 2: One Task a Day.
Post a list of necessary cleaning tasks on your refrigerator. Do one task each day. This is a good approach for people who don't like routines.

Plan 3: 30 Minutes a Day.

Tend to put off weekly chores? Spend 30 minutes each day on one room or one whole-house cleaning task. One possible daily schedule:

Day 1 Kitchen

Day 2 Bathroom

Day 3 Living room, family room, or dining room

Day 4 Bedrooms

Day 5 Office, den, entryways

Day 6 Laundry room

Day 7 Rest

Or you could arrange a task-oriented schedule, like dusting and polishing the furniture in every room one day, for example.

If you are short on time or energy, pick the jobs that are MOST IMPORTANT to you and do them well.

You can **deep clean** your home once or twice a year. Or you can break up that really big job into smaller monthly jobs by deep cleaning room by room.

Once a month, plan to do a thorough cleaning of one room. In a bedroom, for example, you might wash the walls, windows, curtains, floors, and bedding. You might also declutter and organize the closets and drawers. When all the rooms have been cleaned, start over with the first room.

make a plan

Try these proven tips for getting the job done faster and more efficiently:

- Remove clutter from floors and other surfaces before you start cleaning.

- Clean from top to bottom. Start with the cobwebs near the ceiling. Then dust the ceiling fans, tops of bookcases, and other higher-up surfaces. Work your way down. Clean the floors last.

- Instead of removing everything from surfaces, move everything to the right to clean the left side, and vice versa.

- After spraying on a cleaning product, wait a few minutes to allow the product to do its job.

- Try not to get distracted when you are cleaning.

- **Clean each room in a clockwise direction, starting from the door.**

- **Take shortcuts. Let dishes air-dry. Look for furnishings and clothes that resist stains and are easy to clean and care for.**

- **Don't make work. Don't waste time washing an entire wall if all you really need to do is spot-clean. If your clothes aren't noticeably dirty after one use, wear them an extra time.**

- **Do jobs in the same order each time and cleaning will become automatic.**

- **Clean up spills immediately.**

- **Place wastebaskets wherever trash accumulates.**

make a plan

☀ **1** Make housecleaning more **enjoyable** by putting on your favorite music or listening to a book on tape.

☀ **1** Motivate yourself with a **reward** for your cleaning efforts, such as relaxing afterward in a hot tub, watching your favorite TV show, going out to the movies, or reading a book or magazine after cleaning.

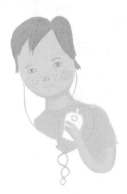

make a plan

The simplest way to cut your cleaning time is to prevent dirt and dust from accumulating:

- Place doormats inside and out.

- Institute a "no shoes" rule for your house.

- Use paint with mold inhibitor added when refinishing the walls.

- Ban food from bedrooms.

- On your kitchen and children's walls, use semigloss rather than flat paint.

- Choose a carpet with built-in stain resistance for high-traffic areas, like hallways.

- Shower with glycerin soap to reduce soap-scum buildup.

make a plan

❶ Research shows that women with children spend more time cleaning than everyone else. The antidote is to enlist the help of family members, because the fastest way to get chores done is to **divide the work** among household members.

❶ Your partner may not mind doing a chore you absolutely hate, and vice versa. However, if your partner doesn't do a job quite the way you would do it yourself, don't make the mistake of criticizing! It helps to have a standard you can agree on, and like many other things in a **partnership,** this may require some compromise.

If you live in a household full of people, you may have extra cleaning challenges — but you also have EXTRA HANDS to help out.

Chores provide an opportunity for family members to spend time together. Whenever possible, make cleaning time a **group activity.** At the very least, do a chore together occasionally.

☀ ❶ Even small children can help clean. For example, while one family member is vacuuming, younger siblings can follow along behind, cleaning baseboards with socks on their hands. Make it a contest to see whose sock puppet gets dirtiest.

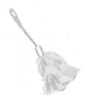

make a plan

Here's what you can reasonably expect from children at various stages of development:

- **Children 3 to 5 years old** can pick up toys and help clear the table. Children at this age generally enjoy "helping" and imitating their parents in other tasks as well.

- **Children 6 to 8 years old** can clear and set the table, empty the garbage, put away clean clothes, feed pets, and pull weeds in the garden.

- **Children 9 to 11 years old** can wash and dry dishes, load and empty the dishwasher, sort laundry, help wash the car, and do simple yard work.

- **Teenagers** can do laundry and other regular housekeeping chores as well as yard work.

Make a **list** of the chores that need to be done regularly. Hold a meeting to talk about each family member's role. Outline daily responsibilities and expectations.

Children of all ages may need some gentle reminders about doing their chores: a posted checklist, notes, or verbal reminders.

Tie **privileges** to getting work done. Offer children a per-job salary or weekly allowance as an incentive, or schedule family outings to the park, beach, or mountains for after the team has completed its goals.

make a plan

Try the following three methods for doling out household responsibilities:

1. Write a chore list every Saturday morning. Have family members write their names next to the chores they will do. If they don't volunteer for something, sign them up.

2. Make a list of chores that need to be done daily or weekly. Then assign chores to each family member for one week. At the end of the week, rotate the schedule.

3. Write jobs on slips of paper and assign a wage or points for each job. Put these slips of paper in a jar. One night a week, have each family member draw a chore.

Teaching children to pick up after themselves is a lesson in PERSONAL RESPONSIBILITY that will follow them into their adult lives.

make a plan

① **Teach** children to take out only a few toys at a time. If they already have two or three toys out, they must put one away before they can take out another. Consider restricting toys to one room of the house.

Younger children will need to be supervised as they learn to do their chores, to understand what constitutes "done," and to be shown appreciation for their help. This will help them see the **value** of their contribution to the family.

Try some of these strategies for making pickup fun:

- Set a laundry basket under a basketball hoop and let kids go for three-pointers.

- Set a timer for 30 seconds and see who can pick up the most stuff before the bell goes off.

- Play a 15-minute game of pickup. Players take up positions in the first room. When you blow the whistle, players start picking up and putting things away. When that room looks good, blow the whistle again and yell out the name of the next room. Wrap up the game with praise for a job well done and a special team reward at the end, such as a bowl of popcorn and a movie.

More and more working people and dual-income families are hiring **outside cleaning help.** If you can afford it, instead of coming home from work to housework, you can spend your free time on activities that are more important to you, or simply rest, relax, and recharge.

❶ The best way to find a professional housecleaner is to ask around.

❶ Be sure to ask for **references.** It's important that you feel comfortable with the person or persons you are hiring to come into your home.

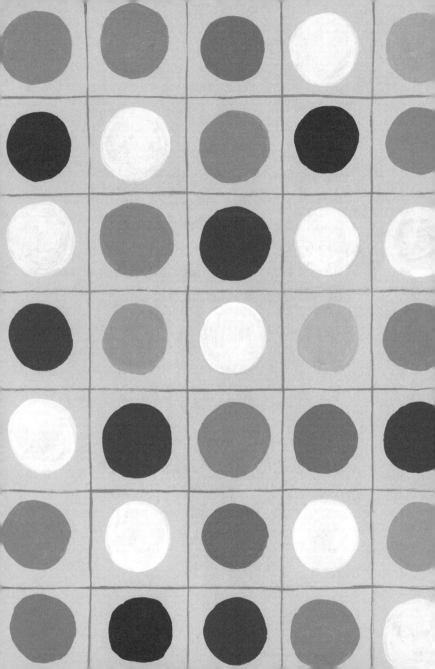

CHAPTER 2

Go Room by Room

Every room in the house presents the challenge of cleaning floors, walls, and windows. And in most homes, clutter knows no boundaries. Less clutter makes cleaning a whole lot easier. Think about it: all that stuff you no longer need or want collects dust and grime. Once you clear out and learn to manage the clutter, you can get down to the business of cleaning floors, walls, and windows with no obstacles to slow you down — and that means progress.

Even if you manage to keep your home clean, it just doesn't look clean when papers and things are piled up on tables, counters, and floors. If you have a lot of **clutter,** it will be well worth your time to purge your home of those things that are simply taking up space.

1 Just because you bought it or someone bought something for you doesn't mean you have to keep it forever.

1 Give yourself **permission** to give away those things that no longer suit your tastes or lifestyle.

Following are five ways to start uncluttering:

- **Make an uncluttering appointment with yourself and honor it.**

- **Unclutter one shelf, drawer, or small area until you are done.**

- **Plan little rewards for getting things done. Example: "I am going to unclutter my kitchen counter, and then I am going to read a magazine for a half hour."**

- **Find a simple solution to one frustrating thing. For example, if it takes you 10 minutes to find a set of earrings each morning, organize your jewelry.**

- **Set a timer or play your favorite CD. When the timer bell rings or your CD stops playing, it's quitting time.**

When cleaning a drawer or shelf or closet, sort the items into five categories:

1. Things you love and/or use.

2. Things you could give away.

3. Things that belong in the trash.

4. Things you could sell.

5. Things that belong elsewhere.

Take items that don't belong where you've found them to their new or proper homes.

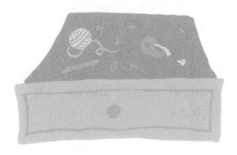

Put new **photos** into an album instead of adding them to the pile that's been accumulating for the past 10 years. Even if you never get around to organizing the backlog, at least your most current photographs will be organized from today forward.

☀ Sort your new **mail** every day; immediately toss anything that is junk.

☀ Resist the urge to just put something down at the spot where you happen to be when you are finished with it; instead, take a moment to put things where they belong.

❶ Change one thing, such as what you do with your bills when they arrive in the mail. Instead of leaving them on the counter, where they are bound to get lost in the paper shuffle, create a folder or large envelope labeled "Bills," and put all your bills into it as they arrive.

❶ Wherever you start uncluttering, plan to tackle the most visible clutter first and work your way into the out-of-sight areas.

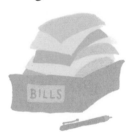

Tips to help you let go of material possessions:

- Instead of picking up each object as you try to decide what to do with it, have someone else hold it. Holding it emphasizes your attachment.

- The more you have, the more you have to take care of. Make a conscious decision to let someone else take over the caretaker job.

- If you get stuck trying to decide whether to keep a particular item or not, set it aside for a day. If you're undecided about what to do with a particular item, it's probably something you could give away, throw away, or sell.

When uncluttering,

it helps to realize that

the most IMPORTANT

THINGS in life are

not things.

A really simple way to find a new home for **reusable items** is to post them on an online bulletin board such as Freecycle. Join your local freecycling community by signing up at www.freecycle.org. Then you can send an e-mail to other members offering the items you wish to give away.

Rather than add to the landfill, **recycle** things you don't need, such as plastic grocery bags and wire hangers. You can also recycle used ink and laser cartridges through the manufacturer, office supply stores, and school fundraising programs.

One time-proven way to get rid of unwanted stuff, and make a few bucks in the process, is to hold a garage or **yard sale.** Invite friends and family members to join you, with the understanding that they do all their own pricing and setup, that they help you on the day of the sale, and that they take all unsold items with them when they leave.

① To **encourage your children** to declutter their rooms, offer to let them keep whatever they make from selling their unwanted items at a garage sale.

go room by room

The key to getting organized is to find the best possible place to store all your things:

- Use a magnetic knife holder mounted on a cabinet door as a home for nail clippers, tweezers, and scissors.

- Hat boxes, tins, and woven baskets contain clutter on shelves while adding to the room's decor.

- Label diaper-wipe containers and use them to store first-aid supplies, makeup, pain relievers, and vitamins.

- Liquor cartons with interior dividers store dry umbrellas or rolled-up artwork.

- Keep a basket at the bottom of the stairs for collecting items that need a lift up.

Uncluttering is half the battle. ORGANIZING is the other half. Without organizing, uncluttering is a job you'll have to do over and over again.

❶ Don't be afraid to **ask for help** if you need it. For example, when you get ready to clean out your closet, invite a friend to help you determine what does and does not look good on you.

❶ Learn to say "no thanks" to things you don't want or need.

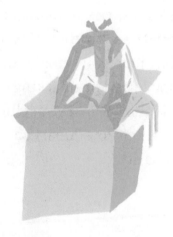

In January of each year, clean out your filing cabinet to make room for the new year's files. Save only **what you need** to save for legal or financial reasons, and discard the rest. Throughout the year, as you file papers, flip quickly through the folder to see whether it contains any papers that can be tossed.

1 The easiest way to maintain a **clutter-free home** is this: for every one item you bring in the front door, send one packing out the back door. When your child receives a new toy, donate an old one to charity.

Following are some simple everyday strategies for taking care of the little things:

- Designate a "drop off" box for library books and videos that need to be returned.

- Keep a "put away" basket in a central location.

- Keep just a few plastic shopping bags and empty margarine and yogurt containers. Recycle all others.

- Think twice about buying things that require extra upkeep, such as knickknacks that have to be dusted and clothing with special washing instructions.

- Simplify. Make a conscious decision to surround yourself only with things you love and use.

With clutter removed from the room you want to clean, you can see the work that needs to be done. Thanks to gravity, **floors** are pretty much an everyday cleaning challenge, while walls and windows are more of a once- or twice-a-year endeavor. But most floors require only regular vacuuming or a light cleaning with a mild solution to keep them looking good.

Tips for keeping hardwood floors clean and glowing:

- Sweep or dust mop often. Use a wool dust mop to shine.

- Vacuum as often as you vacuum carpets. Be sure to use the hard-floor attachment, not the carpet beater brush.

- Damp-mop polyurethaned floors occasionally with a wrung-out mop. Buff waxed floors occasionally to renew shine. Rewax them annually with a wood cleaning/waxing compound.

- Use a white cloth moistened with acetone or nail polish remover to remove oil, paint, marker, lipstick, ink, or tar. Harden candle wax or chewing gum messes with ice and then gently scrape it away with a plastic scraper, such as a credit card.

Mop **wood laminate** floors with a mixture of 1 cup of vinegar in 1 gallon of warm water, or with just plain water. As with hardwood floors, wring out your mop so it is only slightly damp.

☼ If you're not sure whether you have a waxed or polyurethane-coated wood floor, sprinkle a few drops of water on the floor. If the water beads up, the floor is probably coated with polyurethane.

Do not use AMMONIA on any surface if you recently used liquid chlorine bleach or a product containing any bleach.

Mop **ceramic tile, slate, or stone floors** weekly with a cleaner made for ceramic floors or a mixture of 1 cup of vinegar in 1 gallon of water. Do not use detergent or soap, which can dull the surface.

To remove surface stains from **grout,** rub the grout with a piece of folded sandpaper or a pink pencil eraser. For tougher stains, mix 1 tablespoon of bleach with 16 ounces of warm water in a spray bottle. Spray the bleach mixture onto the grout and use a toothbrush to scrub between the tiles.

Vacuum vinyl or **linoleum floors** and remove any spots before wet-mopping. You can remove a scuff-mark with an art-gum or pink pencil eraser. Mop new flooring with warm water only or a mixture of 1 cup of white vinegar in 1 gallon of water. Avoid using detergents or other cleaners that leave a sticky residue that actually attracts dirt.

To clean older linoleum or **vinyl floors,** try mopping with 2 cups of ammonia in 1 gallon of hot water. Use a nylon-bristle brush to lift dirt buildup from grooves and dimples in the flooring. Follow up with a coat or two of acrylic floor wax to help keep the floor clean.

Vacuum carpets at least once a week. About 85 percent of the soiling in carpets is loose dirt. Frequent **vacuuming** will help prevent that dirt from becoming ground in and will extend the life of your carpets. The other 15 percent is oily, sticky stain that vacuuming can't remove. That's why it's important to deep-clean wall-to-wall carpeting every 12 to 18 months.

① Remove **solid soils** from carpet spills by gently scraping the material off with a spatula. Absorb wet spills by blotting them with white paper or cloth towels.

For older or tougher stains, pour **peroxide** onto the stain and cover it with a wet towel. Apply a hot iron set to "cotton" to the wet towel and hold it in place for 15 to 20 seconds. Repeat over the area to transfer the stain to the towel. Take care not to burn the carpet and be sure to turn your face away from the iron's rising steam.

1 Think twice before reaching for any carpet spot-remover product. If it does not remove the spot, you need to completely rinse the product out of the carpet before trying another **stain-removal** method. Even if the stain comes out with the commercial product, the chemicals in the product tend to attract soil to that spot, making the stain seem to reappear.

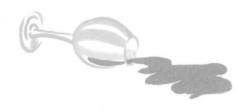

Generally, all you have to do to keep walls looking good is to spot-clean fingerprints, handprints, and smudges on frequently touched spots. Occasionally it may be necessary to clean entire walls:

- Vacuum dust from walls.

- Fill one bucket with two squirts of dishwashing liquid and warm water and another with clean water.

- Begin with a small area at the bottom corner of one wall. Dip a large cellulose sponge in the cleaning solution, squeeze it out, and gently wipe the wall.

- Rinse the area with a second sponge dipped into the clean water and squeezed out.

- Wipe moldings down with a lint-free cloth.

① When washing walls, work from the bottom up to prevent cleanser from streaking dirty sections below.

Spot clean **wallpaper** regularly with a squirt of dishwashing liquid added to a gallon of water. Dip a sponge into the solution, squeeze out the excess water, and wipe away dirt. Rinse with a damp sponge. Blot dry with a lint-free cloth.

MAKE YOUR OWN
Wall Cleaner

Dissolve ½ cup of borax in 1 gallon of warm water. Stir in ½ tablespoon of ammonia.

Three Solutions to Crayon Marks on Walls

1. Dampen a clean cloth with water and dip it in baking soda. Use the cloth to wipe the area firmly to remove the marks. This may take a little "elbow grease."

2. Spray the marks with **WD-40** lubricant and wipe in a circular motion with a clean cloth. Wash away any remaining residue with a sponge wetted with dishwashing liquid and water.

3. Wet an eraser-type cleaning sponge, squeeze out the excess water, and use the sponge to wipe away the marks. This is by far the easiest, most effective solution.

In an IDEAL WORLD,
windows get cleaned —
inside and out — once
or twice a year.

Follow these window-cleaning steps for professional results:

1. Outdoors, sweep the windows, tracks, and sills with a broom. Indoors, vacuum sills and frames.

2. Dip a cloth into the cleanser. Squeeze it out gently. Wash the windows, using circular strokes, working from the outside in.

3. Wipe the glass with a squeegee, paper towels, newspaper, or a lint-free cloth. Use vertical strokes on the outside of the window and horizontal strokes inside. This makes it easier to see if any streaks are on the inside or outside.

4. Wipe away drips around the edges with a dampened chamois cloth or let them air-dry.

5. Dry the windowsill with a rag.

1 Avoid washing windows on a sunny day. If they dry too quickly, they are likely to streak.

MAKE YOUR OWN
Grandpa's Best Window-Washing Formula

½ cup sudsy ammonia (a formulation with a small amount of added detergent)

1 pint rubbing (70 percent isopropyl) alcohol

1 teaspoon dishwashing liquid

Combine the three ingredients in a bucket. Add enough water to make 1 gallon of liquid that will make for the cleanest windows you've ever had.

Clean **window treatments** once a year. Vacuum heavy drapes with an upholstery attachment and lighter drapes with the dusting brush attachment. Wash sheer curtains in the washing machine on the delicate cycle; hang them while still damp, to prevent wrinkles.

Dust horizontal **blinds** regularly. When a buildup needs to be removed, extend the blinds fully and turn the slats to the closed position. Wipe the slats from top to bottom with a slightly damp microfiber cloth, sponge, vacuum brush attachment, or lamb's-wool duster. Then open and reclose the slats in the opposite direction and repeat.

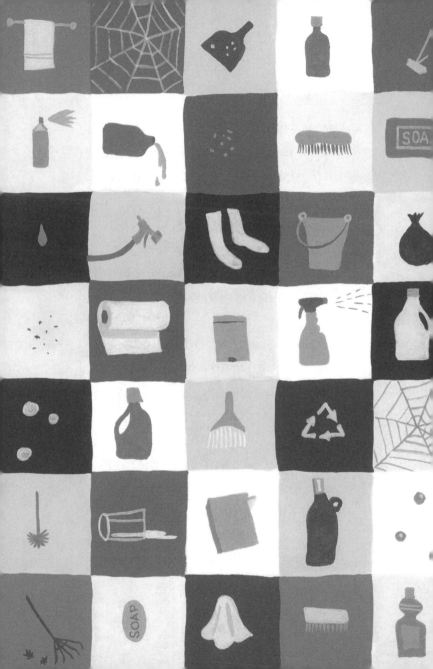

CHAPTER 3

Polish Public Spaces

High-traffic areas in your home — the entryway, family room, living room, and den — get regular use. These are places where household members play, relax, pass through, and drop off their stuff. Regular use means regular cleaning is required.

In the kitchen, food is prepared and eaten, families gather and share the details of their lives, and guests are informally entertained. It is the heart of the home and, like all hearts, it needs extra care to keep it healthy.

The kitchen is the most challenging room to keep clean. There's everyday clutter to contend with, as well as grease, crumbs, and spills. But it's what you can't see that really creates a challenge in the kitchen — bacteria. Your floor may be shiny and your cupboards organized, but a truly clean kitchen requires **daily diligence against germs.**

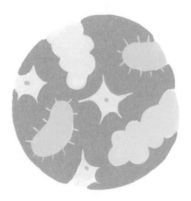

You can get rid of 99 percent of germs with soap and hot water, but you need to disinfect surfaces to kill the germs.

To **disinfect surfaces,** wipe with a liquid chlorine bleach solution (1 tablespoon of bleach in 1 gallon of water), a disinfectant kitchen cleaner, or a nontoxic mist of vinegar, followed by a mist of 3 percent hydrogen peroxide. Let the spray sit for a few minutes, wipe away, and air-dry.

Disinfect everything that comes in contact with raw eggs, meat, poultry, or fish, including your hands, cutting boards, countertops, faucets, utensils, and plates. Before disinfecting, use paper towels to wipe up raw egg and raw meat, fish, or poultry juices, and then discard the towels.

❶ It's a good idea to use a designated sponge for washing dishes and wiping counters that have come in contact with raw meat or eggs, to avoid cross-contamination.

❶ Disinfect used sponges and dishcloths daily.

The best thing you can do to keep countertops **CLEAN** is to keep them **DRY.** Bacteria are everywhere, and they love moist environments.

If you wipe down a surface contaminated by germs, the cloth itself will contaminate other areas when used again. Here are three disinfecting methods:

1. Place damp sponges and cloths in the microwave oven, and "cook" them on high power for 1 minute.

2. Soak sponges for 5 minutes in a dishpan containing a solution of 1 cup of liquid chlorine bleach and 1 gallon of water. Rinse them with clean water and hang to dry.

3. Launder sponges and dishcloths using the hot-water cycle of your washing machine and dry them in the dryer. Toss sponges and dishcloths in the dishwasher with a load of dishes.

polish public spaces

☀ You may be able to remove **ink stains** on your countertop with a splash of rubbing alcohol. To remove countertop **rust stains,** make a paste of baking soda and vinegar and rub it gently into the stain.

To clean dirty grout, pour 3 percent hydrogen peroxide on stained grout seams and cover the area with a towel; let sit overnight.

☀ Freshen upp your **garbage disposal** by grinding citrus fruit rinds with ice cubes and running water.

Simple organizing tips for the kitchen:

- Move items you use infrequently to the backs of cupboards.

- Put out a decorative bowl or basket to collect odds and ends.

- Pare down kitchenware to those things you have used within the past year.

- Organize pantry items by category: pastas, cereals, canned fruits, baking items, and so on.

- Hang a cork bulletin board inside your pantry or a cupboard door; use it to pin up notes, emergency telephone numbers, shopping lists, and stray coupons.

- Create a three-ring binder for storing recipes.

Clean your **stainless-steel sink** with a sudsy nylon sponge. Then rinse it and wipe it dry. Do not use steel wool, abrasive cleansers, ammonia, or bleach, which can damage the finish of the sink. If you need additional cleaning power, wet the sink, sprinkle it with baking soda or another nonabrasive scouring powder, and rub it gently with a sponge.

To **sanitize** your sink, use a commercial disinfectant, a solution of 1 part liquid chlorine bleach to 16 parts of water (except if you have a stainless-steel sink), or a cloth moistened with white vinegar.

To remove white residue that has formed as a result of water evaporating, line the sink with paper towels and saturate them with white vinegar. Let sit for at least 30 minutes. Scrub the sink with a sudsy nylon-mesh sponge, rinse, and wipe dry.

To clear and refresh your **drains,** pour ½ cup of baking soda followed by 1 cup of white vinegar down the drain. Plug the drain and let it fizz for a few minutes. Rinse with boiling water.

For sink rust stains, try an all-metal polish or stainless-steel cleanser.

Clean your **ceramic sink** with a nonabrasive liquid or cream cleanser. Remove stubborn stains and scuff marks with a sponge soaked in club soda.

To clean your **cast-iron sink,** wet the surface, sprinkle with baking soda, and gently scrub with a nylon scrub-mesh sponge. Use abrasive cleaners only in an attempt to remove stubborn stains, and even then only sparingly.

❶ Remove fingerprints, water spots, and germs from **chrome faucets and fixtures** with a cloth saturated with white vinegar or a disposable kitchen wipe.

There are more GERMS in your kitchen sink than on your toilet seat. Think about that the next time you are about to wash produce in the sink.

Hardwood cutting boards are more hygienic than plastic boards. Knife scars in plastic provide hideouts for bacteria that are nearly impossible to kill. Hardwood absorbs the bacteria, trapping it inside. Any surface bacteria die 3 minutes after the surface is washed and dried.

❶ Wet all-wood **cutting boards,** and then microwave on high for 5 minutes to kill any bacteria they contain inside and out.

Season wood surfaces monthly to prevent stains, odor, and bacteria. Microwave mineral oil for 10 seconds. Wipe the oil on the surface. Wait 6 hours and blot excess.

polish public spaces

Before cleaning inside your refrigerator, toss out any food that is out-of-date. Remove perishables to a cooler and nonperishables to a counter. Wash removable refrigerator parts in hot, soapy water.

Dissolve 2 tablespoons of baking soda in 1 quart of hot water. **Wipe the refrigerator and freezer** walls, shelves, and floor with the solution. Rinse with a cloth dipped in clean water, and then dry. To remove dried-on food residue, soak a towel in the baking-soda solution and lay the towel on top of the food residue. Close the door and let sit for at least 20 minutes and simply wipe it away.

The **best time** to clean the inside of your refrigerator is before you go shopping or when it is more empty than full. Wipe jars and containers before putting them back inside a clean refrigerator.

① Never use liquid chlorine bleach to clean the interior of the refrigerator, as it can damage seals, gaskets, and linings.

① The top of the refrigerator can get very grimy. For easier cleanup, cover the top with **plastic food wrap** or a piece of fabric that you can simply peel off and replace every few months.

☀ Place an open box of baking soda in both the refrigerator and freezer compartments to absorb and **prevent odors.**

Don't forget to clean and sanitize the drip pan at the base of your refrigerator (provided it is removable) to prevent it from becoming a breeding ground for bacteria.

☀ Vacuum **the coils** on the bottom or back of the refrigerator at least once a year to keep the unit operating properly.

Use a toothbrush to dislodge debris from the inside corners of cabinets and drawers. Vacuum up crumbs and then clean with equal parts of vinegar and water or an all-purpose cleanser. Next, dampen a cloth with a mixture of ½ cup of vinegar or ½ cup of liquid oil soap in 1 gallon of warm water and use it to wipe **cabinet and drawer fronts.**

Periodically clean the dishwasher heating element with a cloth dampened with vinegar. Then use the cloth to clean the soap and detergent buildup from the dispenser and spray arms.

Mineral deposit buildup in your coffeemaker can slow down brewing time. Follow these steps to remove minerals and restore the flow rate:

1. Pour 4 cups of white vinegar into the water container.

2. Set the glass carafe (lid in place) on the hot plate.

3. Without a paper filter, snap the filter basket in place and switch on the appliance.

4. Let half of the vinegar flow through. Switch off the appliance and let it sit for 10 minutes. Switch it on again and allow the remainder of the solution to run through.

5. Repeat with a clean vinegar solution as many times as needed.

6. Run two cycles of clean water through the unit to rinse it.

If you start with a clean kitchen, it takes only a FEW MINUTES each day to keep it clean.

1 Steam cleaning is an easy way to loosen food particles stuck to the inside of **your microwave.** Pour 1 cup of vinegar or 2 cups of water into a microwave-safe container (add 1 teaspoon of vanilla extract or slices of lemon to the water for a fresh scent). Microwave on high for 5 minutes and wipe the oven clean.

Clean **large kitchen appliance** surfaces with an all-purpose cleaner, soapy water, or white vinegar. Rinse with a damp cloth. Clean stubborn grime with a paste of baking soda and water.

If something has spilled inside your oven, sprinkle salt on the residue while the oven is still warm. (If the spill is dry, lightly wet the residue first.) When the **oven** cools, use a spatula to scrape up the spill, and then wipe remaining residue with a soapy sponge. You can also pour vinegar on the residue and cover it with a damp towel until it can be removed easily.

❶ To minimize future oven-cleaning ordeals, line the bottom of your oven with **aluminum foil,** and replace it when spills occur.

Oven Care

Use the following steps to clean the inside of the oven, taking care to determine whether or not your oven is self-cleaning:

- **Non-self-cleaning oven.** Clean the door gasket and the area around it with a nylon-mesh sponge and hot, soapy water. To remove large amounts of oven grime, use an oven-cleaning product. Keep in mind that oven cleaners are very potent. Be sure to protect your floor from permanent chemical damage by spreading several layers of newspapers in front of the oven. Wear rubber gloves to protect your skin.

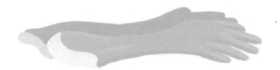

- **Self-cleaning oven.** Use the tips on the previous page to remove burned-on spills. If your racks and broiler pan are silver-colored, remove them and clean as directed below. If they're gray porcelain-coated, they can stay in the oven for the self-cleaning cycle. Once the oven has cooled, use a wet paper towel to wipe up the white residue left behind.

- **Broiler pan and oven racks** can also be cleaned with oven cleaner. Spray them with the product and put them in a trash bag; tie up the bag and leave it outdoors for at least 30 minutes. Remove the pieces from the bag and rinse with a wet sponge. Then wash in hot, soapy water.

To clean your oven **naturally,** wipe off all grease and remove any burned-on food (using tips on page 93). Spritz the oven floor with water, and cover with the contents of one small box of baking soda. Spray the baking soda with enough water to moisten it and let sit overnight, spritzing it again before going to bed. The next day, use a wet sponge to remove the grime.

Use a nylon-mesh sponge and a baking soda and water paste to clean the sides of the oven.

Another way to clean your oven naturally is with **ammonia.** Preheat the oven to 200°F (93°C) and then turn it off. Place a small bowl of ammonia in the oven, close the door, and leave it overnight. The next day, wipe the interior clean with soapy water and a sponge. Use a nylon-mesh sponge to remove baked-on residues.

A grimy **broiler pan** can be sprinkled with detergent while it's hot and then covered entirely with wet paper towels or a dishcloth. Let the pan sit for 30 minutes before washing with hot, soapy water.

The SIMPLEST THING you can do to ease housework is to keep out dirt.

Good-quality **mats** at each entryway, inside and outside, and at the top of basement stairs will greatly reduce the amount of dirt coming in on shoes. During winter or wet weather, consider setting out a boot scraper.

❶ Encourage family members and guests to **remove their shoes** upon entering the house by placing a shoe rack or a basket at each outside door.

❶ Stash a supply of small towels near entryways to wipe your four-footed friends' wet or dirty paws.

polish public spaces

Organizing high traffic areas can go a long way toward making it easier to clean:

- **Keep a basket near the door as a temporary home for borrowed items that need to be returned.**

- **Discourage the dumping of mail, books, and backpacks on the dining room table by setting the table with placemats, dishes, silverware, napkins, and candles.**

- **Organize books, videos, DVDs, and CDs by category.**

- **Store magazines and catalogs in an upright position. They look tidier and it will be easier to find and recycle older issues.**

- **Hide craft projects and other works in progress behind a decorative screen.**

polish public spaces

How often you need to clean every-day living areas depends on how much use they get and what activities take place there.

Everyday cleaning might include a nightly clutter pickup, the folding of throws, the fluffing of pillows, and the spot-cleaning of furniture, carpets, and rugs.

The weekly cleaning routine should include:

- Sweeping away cobwebs
- Dusting all surfaces and displayed objects
- Cleaning and polishing wood furniture
- Vacuuming and mopping

MAKE YOUR OWN
Wood Cleaner & Polish

Mix ½ teaspoon of olive oil and
½ cup of vinegar or lemon juice in
a plastic spray bottle. Shake well.
Spray onto a microfiber or flannel
cloth and use the cloth to clean
and polish wood furniture. The
vinegar or lemon juice cleans the
wood, and the oil lubricates it.

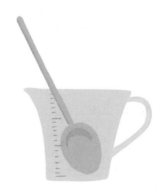

Vacuum **upholstered furniture** with an upholstery attachment. Between vacuumings, remove hair, lint, and food particles with a tape-style lint remover or foam sponge.

Dab **stains** on upholstered furniture immediately with a clean white cloth wetted with lukewarm water. To avoid spreading the stain, work from the outside of the stain inward. If that doesn't work, spray 3 percent hydrogen peroxide on the stain and cover with a towel. Press the towel into the fabric and then allow it to stand for 8 hours or overnight. Repeat as necessary. Spot-clean entire pieces of older **furniture** to avoid creating spotty-looking fabric.

Following are some plain and simple tricks for cleaning other home furnishings:

- Vacuum lampshades with the dusting brush attachment, dust them with a clean paintbrush, or wipe them gently with a foam latex sponge or lint-removal tool.

- Periodically remove the glass casings of ceiling light fixtures and remove dead insects and dirt.

- Wipe the ceiling fan blades with a cloth dampened with white vinegar so that it will cut through grease and dirt.

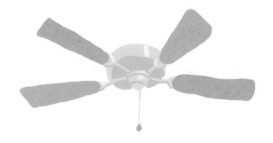

polish public spaces

- Clean the edges of book pages with a natural bristle brush, and clean the covers with a soft cloth. Align books with the outer edge of shelves to avoid dust buildup on those edges.

- Pour some salt into a paper bag and add artificial flowers. Shake vigorously to clean.

- Spray glass cleaner onto a cloth and then wipe the glass and frames of art and photographs.

- Clean soiled candles with an absorbent cotton ball dipped in rubbing alcohol.

- Dust bulbs regularly. Clean bulbs save electricity and last longer because less heat builds up inside them. A dirty light bulb emits 20 percent less light than a clean one.

A **white ring on wood** is likely to be a stain in the wax, not the finish. Try one of these five simple solutions to remove it:

- Rub with a cotton cloth moistened with denatured alcohol.

- Apply a small amount of toothpaste to the spot. Rub with a clean cloth.

- Apply mayonnaise to the stain and rub it in. Let it sit overnight.

- Moisten a cotton swab with saliva and wipe the stain away.

- Rub equal parts of olive oil and white vinegar with a clean cloth. Remove and rewax.

Once a month or so, unplug **your computer** and clean the casing and monitor or the laptop and liquid crystal display (LCD) screen with a microfiber cloth slightly dampened with water. Never apply a cleaning solution directly.

1 Wipe grimy keyboard key tops with a cloth dampened with rubbing alcohol.

At each change of daylight saving time, check and clean **your smoke detectors.** Wipe the outside casing and vacuum the inside. When you're finished cleaning the detector, test it. Once a year, replace the batteries.

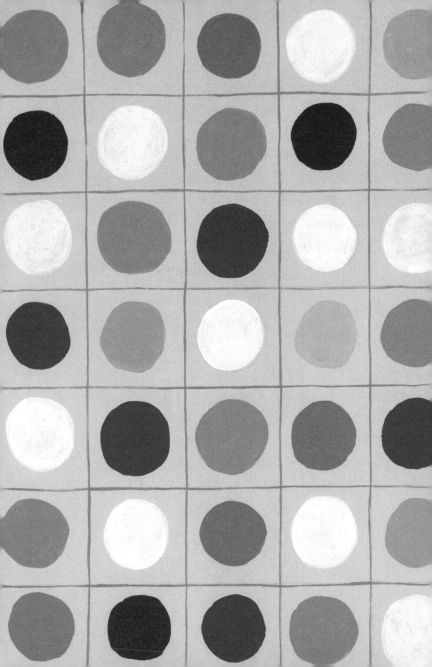

CHAPTER 4

Freshen Private Places

There's nothing like a freshly made bed and sparkling bathroom to help you relax when your time is yours. And if your time mostly belongs to the baby, you know that keeping the nursery clean is important for the well-being of both you and your child.

Some areas of the house are frequently neglected because they are kept behind closed doors. The secret to keeping them neat and tidy is periodic organization and a regular cleaning routine.

Maintain a clean and **cozy bedroom** by developing a cleaning routine. Each morning, put away anything that does not belong in your bedroom. Before going to bed, invest a few moments to put away clothes you will wear again, and put everything else in the hamper or dry-cleaner bag.

1 For a bed that practically makes itself, replace your top sheet and comforter or bedspread with a **duvet and duvet cover.** Just shake the duvet and your bed is made instantly.

Your weekly cleaning routine might include the following activities:

- Straighten the dresser top.

- Put away any clean clothes.

- Dust the wall hangings and other decorations.

- Polish any wood furniture.

- Dust the light bulbs and lampshades.

- Change the sheets (or duvet cover) and pillowcases.

- Wipe down wall switches.

- Shake out any small area rugs.

- Vacuum the floors.

When cleaning the floors, don't forget to clean **under the bed.** Use a dust mop on hard flooring to grab dust balls.

To avoid a pile-up of laundry, consider washing linens and then putting the same set of sheets back on the bed. For variety, switch to a different set when the seasons change.

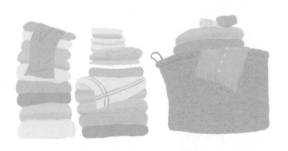

At least once a week,

throw open a window to

FRESHEN THE AIR

in each bedroom.

Bedroom Organizing Tips

- **Provide every bedroom with a laundry hamper and a wastebasket.**

- **Place a decorative bowl or basket on dresser tops to collect loose change and pocket items.**

- **Create storage space with closet shelving, freestanding drawer units, and under-the-bed and over-the-door organizers.**

- **Install hooks in your closet or behind a door for airing worn clothes you will wear again before laundering.**

- **Keep the floor of your closet clear for easy vacuuming.**

- **Periodically take inventory of your closets and drawers; give away or sell anything you no longer love or wear.**

Although the **guest bedroom** may be rarely used, it still needs to be cleaned. Once a month, toss the bedspread in the dryer for 10 minutes to kill dust mites. Sweep away cobwebs; dust closet shelves, wall hangings, lampshades, and bulbs; polish the furniture; shake out small rugs; and vacuum.

Before visitors arrive, clear space in the closet for their clothing. Leave a set of towels for each guest on the bed. After they leave, strip the bed and wash all the bedding. Vacuum the mattress and spray it with a fabric refresher. Air out the mattress and remake the bed.

Kids of all ages want their privacy. Let them know that if they keep their rooms cleaned up, you will not have to enter except for periodic, preannounced inspections. Establish a **morning pickup routine** that might include making beds, hanging up towels, and putting away pajamas. The evening routine might include putting away toys and tossing dirty clothes in the hamper.

Depending on their ages, children can also be expected to do some weekly cleaning of their bedrooms, which might include dusting or vacuuming. If you give children cleaning products to use, be sure to supervise them.

The trick to getting kids to stay organized is to make it easy:

- **A shoe bag hung low on the back of a door can be used to store small toys.**

- **Gather stuffed animals in a nylon hammock hung up in one corner. Or hang colored ribbon horizontally between two hooks. Use clothespins to clip on small stuffed animals or artwork.**

- **Store toys and games on shelves with bins rather than in toy boxes.**

- **Install kid-height wall pegs for book bags, pajamas, and clothes.**

- **Increase drawer space with slide-out drawers under children's beds.**

- **Label shelves, drawers, and containers. For toddlers, label with drawings, photographs, or pictures cut out of magazines.**

freshen private places

Suggestions for the care and cleaning of linens:

- **Always launder new linens.**

- **Fabric softener decreases towel absorbency. Use only monthly.**

- **Avoid liquid chlorine bleach to whiten sheets; it will eventually cause sheets to yellow.**

- **Store a set of sheets between the mattress and the box spring — ready for a quick change.**

- **Use a mattress pad for comfort, mattress protection, and to reduce the presence of dust mites.**

- **Wash pillows on the gentle cycle and run them through the rinse and spin cycles twice.**

- **Add two clean tennis balls when drying feather pillows and down comforters to fluff.**

The best defense against

DUST MITES and

other allergens is a good

offense. Clean bedrooms,

bedding, and closets

frequently to keep dust

mites under control.

The **bathroom** has developed a reputation for being the nastiest room in the house when it comes to cleaning. But it doesn't have to be that way. There are some very simple things you can do every day to virtually stop bacteria, mold, and mildew in their tracks.

☀ Use a daily "no-wipe" shower cleaner to prevent soap-scum buildup. **Squeegee** doors and walls after each shower to discourage mold. Use an exhaust fan or open a window while showering to vent the moist air.

☀ Hang towels so they will dry as quickly as possible.

freshen private places

Wipe the sink, faucets, and counter-top after the final use every morning.

Use a flush-release cleaning product in the toilet bowl. Or brush the bowl daily to keep it clean.

❶ Pour all-purpose cleaner in the toilet-brush holder to **keep it fresh** and ready for use.

❶ Keep sanitizing wipes on hand for cleaning on the fly.

Once a week, give your bathroom a more thorough **top-to-bottom** cleaning. Use a diluted solution of all-purpose cleaner or a commercial bathroom cleaner to clean sinks, counters, and shower stalls.

❶ Use separate sponges or cleaning cloths for cleaning the toilet area, which is likely to have the highest concentration of germs.

❶ Avoid storing toothbrushes near the toilet. With every flush, particles of water (and *E. coli* germs) can spray and land up to 20 feet away. Always close the toilet lid before flushing.

☀ If you prefer to do bathroom cleaning on a **"catch-as-catch can"** basis, try cleaning the toilet, sink, and mirror while supervising children in the bathtub.

☀ Using the nontoxic product below, you can clean the shower while you are in it. Scrub the walls and floor, and then scrub yourself (but not with the shower cleanser!).

MAKE YOUR OWN
Tub and Tile Cleaner

Combine ¼ cup of borax and ¼ cup of baking soda. Add 1½ cups of hot water and stir until mixed. Apply, scrub, and rinse.

Ideas to help with the most daunting bathroom challenges:

- **Erase stains in the toilet or on any porcelain surface with a pumice stick.**

- **Scrub mold and mildew with a few drops of dishwashing liquid in warm water. Then scrub with 1¼ cup of liquid chlorine bleach in 1 quart of water. Wait 20 minutes and repeat.**

- **Except for on grout, spray distilled white vinegar onto mold. Let vinegar sit, without rinsing.**

- **Periodically wash plastic shower liners in the washing machine with hot water and detergent on the regular cycle. Throwing in a bath towel helps scrub mildew and soap scum off the liner.**

freshen private places

To keep the **nursery** and baby equipment healthy, it's important to clean and disinfect surfaces that are likely to become contaminated with diapering activity residuals, including toys that children put in their mouths, crib rails, the diaper-changing table, and the diaper pail.

After use, remove the **high-chair tray** and scrub it in warm, sudsy water. Rinse and dry. Every few days, use a toothbrush to clean out crevices in the chair. Wash all other parts with a hot, soapy sponge. Then wipe surfaces with hydrogen peroxide and air-dry.

Use a handheld vacuum to clean crevices and recesses of **car seats** and **baby strollers.** Clean the bodies with warm, soapy water and wipe dry.

Periodically, use a sponge and warm, soapy water to clean the **portable play yard.** Disinfect with hydrogen peroxide.

❶ Wash plastic **teething rings and toys** in the top rack of your dishwasher or by hand in hot, soapy water. Disinfect after illness or sharing with other children by wiping with hydrogen peroxide. Launder washable soft toys as needed.

Babies are at higher risk with exposure to chemicals than adults are because their skin, respiratory, and gastrointestinal absorption of toxic materials is greater than that of adults.

MAKE YOUR OWN
Natural Cleaner and Sanitizer

Mix 15 drops of grapefruit seed extract (GSE) with 2 cups warm water. Pour the solution into a spray bottle. Spray the area with the GSE solution and let sit for at least 15 seconds to air-dry. Wipe the area dry.

Formula courtesy of Pure Liquid Gold

The most effective defense against the spread of illness is frequent HAND WASHING, especially after using the bathroom, diapering the baby, and before preparing or eating food.

freshen private places

If you are using a plastic pad on your **changing table,** swab it with a disinfectant wipe after each diaper change. Remove and wash cloth pad covers as often as needed. Disinfect the table surface with a diluted bleach solution after soiling.

❶ Always empty solid waste from disposable diapers into the toilet and flush. Fold up the diaper, with the soiled side in the center, and toss it in the trash or a diaper pail.

❶ Sprinkle baking soda liberally into the diaper, the trash can, or diaper pail after each deposit, to prevent odors.

Diaper Duty

Prewash cloth diapers with laundry detergent in cold water on the presoak cycle to remove soiling without setting stains. Then wash the load in hot water on the longest cycle with a cold-water rinse. Following are some washing options and cautions:

- Fragrance-free detergent is recommended for baby items.

- Add ½ cup of baking soda to the wash to help whiten and soften diapers (when you add baking soda, you can use less detergent).

- You can use bleach occasionally to sanitize and whiten, but regular use will weaken the fabric.

- Fabric softener will reduce the diapers' absorbency, so use it only occasionally.

freshen private places

- An alternative to fabric softener is white vinegar; use ½ cup in the rinse cycle, but avoid using vinegar in a load with diaper covers, as it will reduce the covers' waterproofing. Always follow the instructions on the care label for diaper covers.

- Put the diapers in the dryer on the high heat setting for 60 minutes or until they're completely dry. Machine drying helps sterilize the diapers. You could also dry the diapers in direct sunlight, which also sterilizes them. Then run an empty wash cycle with bleach to disinfect your washer before the next load.

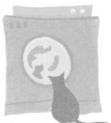

❶ If you use a cloth-diaper pail liner, own two of them, so you always have a clean one available when the other is in the wash.

Wash all **new baby clothes** and diapers before you use them, to remove chemical residues. To preserve fire-retardant qualities, launder baby clothing in detergent, not soap.

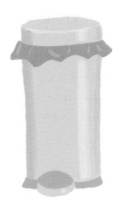

For Safety's Sake

- Keep the floors where your baby plays as clean as possible.

- Keep the diaper pail locked to keep toddlers out.

- Always make sure you have good ventilation when cleaning around your baby. When disinfecting with bleach, do so when the baby is in another room, and open a window.

- When cleaning up body fluids, such as blood, vomit, or feces, you should wear rubber gloves and wash your hands afterward.

- Keep your fingernails short and wash your hands often to lessen the chance of spreading germs.

freshen private places

Did someone have an "accident"? It happens on occasion. When it does, prevent lingering urine odors on your mattress by following these steps:

1. Dampen the "accident" area with a clean, wet cloth.

2. Sprinkle the dampened area with borax detergent.

3. Use the wet cloth to thoroughly scrub the area.

4. Allow the area to dry, and then vacuum up the residue.

Keep all cleaning products OUT OF THE REACH **of toddlers. Ingestion could be lethal!**

Basements and attics accumulate more than their fair share of junk, but these rooms only need periodic cleaning. The **laundry room,** on the other hand, should be a regular stop when you're cleaning the rest of your home.

Store laundry detergent and other products in cabinets, on shelves, or in a freestanding cart. Shelf liners can be sponged down to remove dust and grime. To keep the laundry room floor clear, hang the ironing board on a wall or the back of a door, and instead of a traditional clothes rack for air-drying, consider a foldable wall unit.

freshen private places

Monthly, clean the lid and top of the **washing machine** with equal parts of white vinegar and water. In a sink, pour a little of the vinegar/water solution into fabric softener and bleach dispensers. Scrub these containers with an old toothbrush and rinse.

☀ Clean washer tub of residuals by running a hot-water cycle with 2 cups of white vinegar.

☀ If possible, set up a laundry **pretreatment area** away from the washer and dryer, since many soil- and stain-removal products can damage the finish and control panels of these appliances.

freshen private places

Clean the dryer lint trap after each load. Once a year, clean the dryer as follows:

- Remove the lint trap and use a vacuum attachment to remove all the accumulated lint from under the lint trap.

- Pull the washer and dryer out from the wall and vacuum the machines' backs and the floor.

- Clean the exhaust duct: unplug the dryer, disconnect the duct, vacuum, and reconnect.

- Turn on the dryer, then head outside to check that the inside flaps of the exhaust hood move freely. If your hood points downward, hold a mirror under the hood to get a good look.

- Every year or so, have the dryer cleaned by a qualified technician.

Clean the soleplate, or the bottom of your **iron,** to remove the mineral buildup that can stain fabric. Wipe the cool soleplate with a sudsy cloth. Remove corrosion with a cloth saturated in white vinegar.

If the soleplate holes seep **mineral deposits,** the reservoir of your iron needs cleaning. Fill the reservoir one-quarter full with white vinegar, and steam iron a towel until the reservoir is empty. Repeat if necessary. Rinse with distilled water. Iron with distilled water only to prevent buildup and always empty the water into the sink while it is still hot to dry out the reservoir.

freshen private places

The hardest part of cleaning and organizing a **basement,** an **attic,** or a **garage** is getting started. Schedule a family cleanup day. Or set aside 30 to 60 minutes each week for your storage-organizing project. Sort things into categories:

Donations — unspoiled things that someone else might use

For-Sale Items — things you can sell at a yard sale or consignment shop

Trash — anything worn-out or broken and not worth fixing

Keepers — anything you have used recently or that you truly love

Put the trash items out with your regular garbage pickup, unless they fall into the category of household **hazardous waste.** In addition to many cleaning supplies, other hazardous waste items include:

- Paint and paint thinner
- Motor oil and gasoline
- Antifreeze
- Brake and transmission fluids
- Car batteries

❶ Check with your local household hazardous waste collection program to find out how to properly dispose of these items. Some communities offer an annual collection service.

Simple Storage Tips

- Base decisions about what to store where on the level of accessibility required.

- Limit attic storage to things you need only occasionally, such as holiday decorations and tax records.

- Sort and then store like items (sports equipment, tools, memorabilia) together.

- For easy stacking, buy tubs that are all the same size, and label.

- Use lidded storage tubs rather than cardboard boxes to keep out pests and moisture.

- In the basement, keep storage boxes high and dry on sturdy shelves or pallets.

- Cover large items with sheets or tarps to keep off the dust.

PART TWO

Challenges Inside and Out

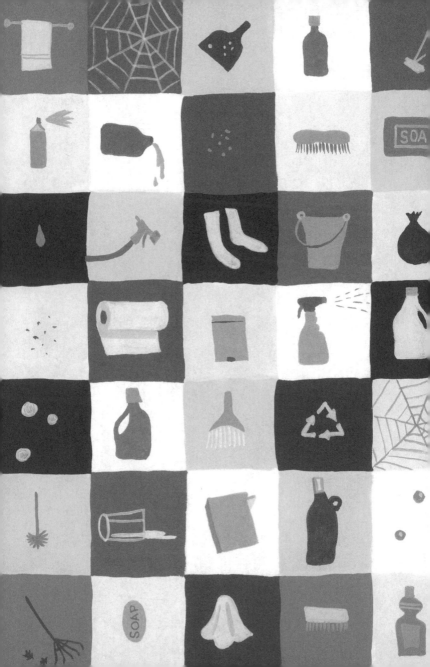

CHAPTER 5

Clothes & Accessories

Ever had a day when you *didn't* come into contact with a personal item that needed cleaning? Probably not. Every day we face the challenges of dirty shoes, dirty clothes, and dirty eyeglasses. In most households, laundry is the biggest challenge. But everyday cleaning also means taking good care of everything from luggage to jewelry. If you've ever wondered how to launder lingerie or remove mildew from leather, you'll find answers to these dilemmas and more in the following pages.

Laundry is one of those chores that can seem endless, especially in large households. No sooner do you finish a **load of wash** than you have another to do. There's probably not much you can do about that. But you can take steps to make the whole process more efficient.

❶ Assign a **laundry basket** to each family member. Have each individual use his or her basket to bring dirty laundry to the laundry room and also to return clean clothes to his or her room.

clothes & accessories

Presort dirty clothes into the three major types of wash loads: **whites, lights, and darks.** Next, sort by fabric type and degree of soil. Separate delicate items, such as woven knits and sheer fabrics.

❶ The simplest way to sort in the laundry room is using a triple-sorter laundry cart with three large fabric bags that hang from a sturdy metal frame.

Wash **heavily soiled items** separately from everyday items that are lightly soiled. Because soils are deposited in the wash water, washing heavily soiled items with lightly soiled items can make the latter even dirtier!

Wash the delicate items separately. Use the delicate setting on your washer, hand wash and hang them to dry, or have them dry-cleaned.

❶ Do not wash **towels** and fuzzy fleecy fabrics with corduroys and permanent-press garments that attract lint.

Never wash lights and darks together; ONE RED SOCK can turn an entire load of white clothing into pink clothing.

The choice of water temperature depends on the amount of soil, the fabric type, and the colorfastness of fabrics in the wash load:

- A hot water temperature of around 130°F (54°C) is recommended for keeping whites white. You should also use hot water for diapers and heavily soiled clothes.

- Use warm water in the range of 90° (32°C) to 110°F (43°C) to wash fabrics that are light-colored, noncolorfast, permanent press, or moderately soiled.

- Use cold water at a temperature of about 80°F (27°C) or colder to wash lightly soiled loads, dark or bright colors that might fade or bleed, and delicate items, including washable woolens, that may shrink in warm temperatures.

When selecting the **agitation level** of the machine, choose the gentle or hand-wash cycle for delicate fabrics and the permanent-press setting to reduce wrinkling of man-made fabrics. Use normal or regular agitation for all other wash loads.

❶ Do not overload the washer. Shake and drop items loosely into the tub and fill it no more than **three-quarters full.**

Before adding each item to the washer, check to make sure it is wash-ready:

- Pretreat stains and spots.

- Zip zippers and fasten hooks.

- Tie strings and sashes loosely.

- Remove anything in pockets, including lint.

- Remove all unwashable trim-mings, including belts, pins, and buckles.

- Turn down shirt sleeves.

- Turn prints and dark clothing inside out to preserve their color.

- Mend fallen hems and rips.

Feel free to adjust **recommended detergent** measurement as necessary. Use more than the recommended amount for larger loads, heavily soiled clothes, or harder water. Use slightly less than the recommended amount for smaller loads, lighter soiling, or softer water.

① Fabric softener may reduce the effectiveness of flame retardancy in children's sleepwear. Instead of **fabric softener,** add ½ cup of white vinegar to the rinse cycle to help soften clothes and keep colors bright. However, note that vinegar can cause some fading of darker clothes.

Be careful not to wash a freshly stained item in hot water without first attempting to remove the stain. **Heat can set** a fresh stain. Apply detergent pretreatments and then wash garments immediately or rinse it out completely to avoid discoloration.

☀ Keep a stain-removal stick in your purse or glove box to treat protein-based stains as they occur.

☀ Never use **liquid chlorine bleach** in the wash if you plan to use vinegar in the rinse; use oxygen bleach instead. The combination of chlorine and vinegar can create noxious fumes.

Delicate items such as lingerie, or items with a fabric care label that recommends **hand-washing** should not be machine washed. Place these items in a sink basin filled with cool water. Add a capful of dishwashing liquid or a light-duty detergent. Gently squeeze the suds through the fabric and then let the items soak for 10 minutes. Rinse with cool water. Do not wring; instead, lay them flat on a white towel, then roll up the towel and squeeze dry. Unroll the towel and hang the items or lay them flat to dry.

The closer a hamper is to where household members get undressed, the MORE LIKELY it is that dirty clothes will end up in it.

clothes & accessories

If a fabric care label says **Dry Clean Only,** don't wash or even spot clean it! Clothing made of rayon, silk, and wool blends may shrink, change colors, or lose shape.

❶ Always remove dry-cleaned garments from their plastic bags and allow them to air out to avoid breathing the laundering chemical perchloroethylene.

If garments have a *very strong* chemical smell, the item is not dry or not enough of the solvent has been removed. Air out garments for at least a day. If you notice the strong smell frequently, consider a different dry cleaner.

When you take clothes out of the washing machine, closely examine any items that were stained before washing. If the **stain** is still there, treat it again and rewash.

Clean the lint filter before **loading the dryer.** Set aside items that need to be line-dried or dried flat. Use the normal temperature setting for drying cottons and heavier items. Select the permanent-press setting for drying lighter-weight or synthetic fabrics. The low setting is for drying delicates. The air-fluff setting is not intended for drying, but is useful for shaking dust from curtains or for softening fabrics.

clothes & accessories

☀ Avoid overloading the dryer. If clothes have **room to circulate,** they will dry faster and have fewer wrinkles.

☀ To reduce drying time, try adding fabric softener to your rinse cycle when washing.

Need to smooth a load of wrinkled clothes or linens left too long in the dryer? Toss a damp, lint-free towel into the dryer and run it on the low setting for 10 to 15 minutes.

Removing slightly damp clothes from the dryer reduces the need for ironing. These tips may be useful for clothes that do need pressing:

- Start with items that require a low heat setting, such as silk and synthetics, and finish with items that require higher heat.

- For pressing with steam, use distilled water, and pour it into your iron before turning it on.

- Iron smaller areas, such as collars and cuffs, first and larger areas last.

- Spray-on starch makes it easier to iron and provides a crisp finish for heavier fabrics such as cottons.

NEVER leave a dryer running while sleeping or when you leave the house. Lint buildup in the outside vent or a faulty dryer can cause a fire.

Any cosmetic tools that come in daily contact with your skin can become a breeding ground for bacteria. Following are some simple guidelines for keeping all of these tools and your skin clean:

- Wash your eyeshadow applicators, reusable cosmetic sponges, compact sponge and powder puff at least once a week with a mild shampoo and air-dry. Or use a fresh disposable sponge every day.

- Clean the metal pieces and pads of your eyelash curler with a cotton ball dipped in eye-makeup remover.

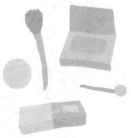

Bath implements also need regular care. Rinse your **loofah sponge** under hot water after every use to flush away dead skin cells and prevent bacteria from growing. Shake it to remove excess water, and hang it to dry outside the shower to avoid mildewing.

To clean your loofah, rinse it in clean water; then soak it in a solution of 1 teaspoon of liquid chlorine bleach and 1 quart of warm water. If possible, let it dry in the sun.

1 Once a week, toss any synthetic **shower puffs** into the washing machine in a hot water cycle.

Taking good care of **hairbrushes** will prolong their life. At least once a week, use a comb to loosen any strands of hair from the brush's bristles. Once a month or so, remove hair and scrub your hairbrush and bristles with a toothbrush dipped into sudsy dishwashing liquid and water. Rinse quickly holding the brush vertically with the handle pointing up and allow it to air-dry on a hard surface, away from sunlight, with the bristles facing down.

1 Do not immerse good-quality, natural-bristle brushes in water. Follow the manufacturer's instructions for best results.

1 Over time, lint will collect in your **blow-dryer,** causing the dryer to overheat. Monthly, unplug the dryer, twist off the grid at the back, and remove the screen. Use a soft toothbrush to brush away dust and hair that has collected on the screen. Then replace the parts.

To clean your **curling iron,** unplug the iron and wipe the outside surfaces with a damp, soapy sponge. Dampen a cotton ball with rubbing alcohol or nail polish remover and use it to swipe the soiled area. Rinse with a water-dampened cotton ball.

Don't save every old toothbrush, but do set aside a few for SPECIAL CLEANING ASSIGNMENTS.

Nine Nifty Uses for Old Toothbrushes

1. Clean out your garlic press.

2. Clean off a hand grater.

3. Brush stain treatments into fabrics before laundering.

4. Gently scour around the base of bathroom and kitchen faucets.

5. Clean your contact lens case.

6. Clean jewelry.

7. Scrub toaster wires and racks.

8. Lift dust from sliding-door tracks.

9. Clean a can opener blade.

❶ It's a good idea to wash old toothbrushes in the dishwasher to clean and disinfect them prior to reuse.

If you wear glasses, follow these steps for **lens care** daily:

1. Immerse the eyeglasses in warm, soapy water.

2. Rub the lenses gently with your fingers.

3. Rinse to wash away dirt and oil.

4. Gently dry the lenses and frames with a soft, lint-free cloth.

❶ Blow dust particles off **camera,** binocular, or other lenses with an ear syringe. Do not use compressed air in a can, which might damage a delicate lens. If the lens appears dirty, breathe on it to create a mist, and then wipe the surface gently with a microfiber cloth or camera-lens-cleaning tissue.

clothes & accessories

Luggage Care

- **Wash hard-sided luggage with warm water and dishwashing liquid. Remove residue with a damp cloth. For stubborn stains, apply rubbing alcohol on the dry surface with a toothbrush.**

- **Toss unconstructed luggage and fabric bags in the washing machine on the delicate cycle, and hang to dry. Spot-clean with a slightly soapy sponge.**

- **Spray smooth leather bags and briefcases with leather protectant at the time of purchase. To clean, apply a cream leather cleaner with a soft cloth.**

- **Vacuum inside of luggage. If musty, wipe the interior with a mixture of one part vinegar and five parts water. Allow the bag to air in the sun.**

Allow **muddy boots and shoes** to air-dry, away from heat and light. Bang the soles and remove dirt from soles and uppers with a stiff nylon brush. Wipe remaining dirt with a damp cloth, and then apply leather cleaner and conditioner.

To remove **white salt lines,** sponge footwear with water and air-dry. If the lines reappear, pour white vinegar on a damp cloth and wipe. Dry with a soft cloth. When the leather is nearly dry, apply leather conditioner to restore the natural moisture.

❶ Always spray new leather shoes with a leather protectant to help prevent stains, and respray them every few weeks.

Got mildew? Here's what to do with mildewed leather or fabric items:

1. Bring the item outdoors and brush off mildew with a dry sponge, cloth, or nylon-bristle brush.

2. Use a sponge dampened with soapy water to wipe clean. Air-dry away from heat and sunlight. If item is leather, apply leather conditioner.

3. If mildew persists, sponge lightly with a mixture of equal parts of rubbing alcohol and water. Lightly wipe again with water only and let air-dry. Finish leather items with a treatment of conditioner.

Preventing Smelly Shoes

- To freshen shoes, place cedar blocks inside or sprinkle liberally with baking soda. (Shake out the baking soda before wearing.)

- Sprinkle salt in canvas shoes to absorb moisture.

- Wipe the insoles and insides with a mixture of one part vinegar and five parts water. Air-dry outside.

- Keep gym bags fresh by placing a fabric softener sheet in each shoe before toting.

❶ Rather than buy an expensive little bottle of shoe **leather cleaner,** buy a larger bottle of leather upholstery cleaner for all your leather belongings.

clothes & accessories

How to wash athletic shoes with canvas, leather, or nylon uppers:

1. Lay down newspaper and fill a dishpan with warm water.

2. Remove insoles. Machine wash shoelaces.

3. Dip one shoe in the water and set on the newspaper.

4. Squirt dishwashing liquid on a nylon scrubbing sponge and scrub the shoe inside and out.

5. Use a toothbrush for stubborn stains. Repeat steps for second shoe.

6. Dip insoles in the water, and scrub with the sponge.

7. Swish shoes and insoles in water to remove soap. Rinse.

8. Stuff the shoes with paper towels and allow to air-dry.

Three solutions for **gum on the shoe:**

1. Place shoe in a plastic grocery bag. Press the sticky portion into the side of the bag. Place the bag, with the shoe inside, in the freezer for at least 1 hour. Remove from the freezer and pull the shoe away from the bag. The gum should stick to the bag.

2. Fill a zippered plastic bag with ice cubes and hold it directly on the gum until it freezes. Pry the gum off the shoe with a putty knife.

3. Spray WD-40 on the gummy area. Wait 1 minute. Then wipe away the gum and the oily spray with a paper towel.

There is no one-fits-all cleaning solution for **jewelry.** What makes diamonds sparkle, for example, would ruin pearls. Ultrasonic cleaners are safe for cleaning all-metal jewelry as well as most diamonds, rubies, emeralds, sapphires, and tourmalines, but it could fracture other gems. Gemstones with adhesive should not be put in an ultrasonic cleaner.

The safest and gentlest way to clean most **gems** is with an old, soft toothbrush dipped in a mild solution of dishwashing liquid in warm water. Check with your jeweler for the best way to clean different pieces.

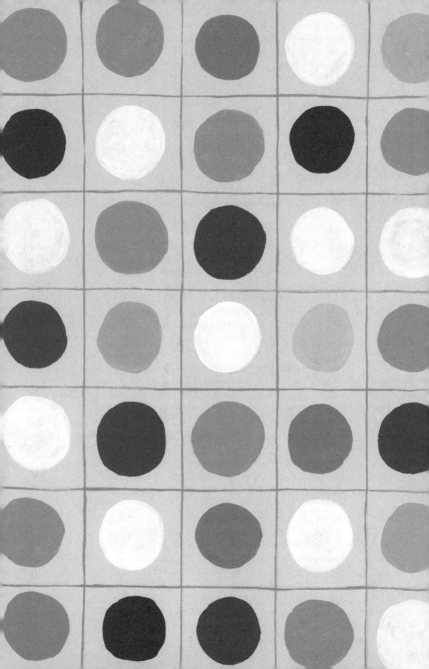

CHAPTER 6

Pets, No Pests

We love our pets. They are friends and family. Unfortunately, they aren't our only animal housemates. Sometimes rodents and insects visit and try to move in permanently. Not only are these pests unwelcome, they litter the home with nests, wastes, and dead bodies — and can leave behind a path of destruction ranging from moth-eaten woolens to structural damage. Luckily, there are ways to minimize the effort it takes to clean up after *all* your critters. And that means more time for fetch!

pets, no pests

Primary care of your pet begins with **feeding and watering.** Whatever type of pet you have, it's important to clean the food and water bowls daily to prevent the buildup of dirt and bacteria.

❶ Place pet bowls on a washable mat or tray to protect your flooring against spills and drips. Wash with hot, soapy water at least once a week or as needed. Disinfect the mat or tray periodically.

To reduce the occurrence of hair-balls vomited up on your furniture and floors, try grooming your cat regularly. There are also cat foods specially formulated to reduce this unpleasant aspect of cat ownership.

1 Pet expert Arden Moore suggests putting a dab of petroleum jelly on your cat's nose; the cat will lick it off and ingest it, which helps move the **hairball buildup** out of the stomach.

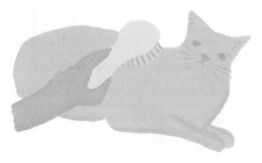

pets, no pests

It's your responsibility to clean up after your pet. **Pet waste** can carry viruses, bacteria, and parasites that are extremely harmful. If your yard has feces in it, just playing ball outside can lead to infection.

☀ When walking your dog, bring along a bag for feces collection.

☀ You can also bury pet waste. Just **dig a hole** at least 5 inches deep, toss in the feces, and fill the hole with dirt. This is a good strategy if you are hiking in the woods, provided you carry a trowel with you.

Picking up after your pet REDUCES THE RISK of disease and keeps the areas where you walk clean.

Pet Waste No-No's

- **Do not dispose of or leave pet waste in a ditch, storm drain, street, sidewalk, or trail. It contributes to the pollution of nearby streams and lakes.**

- **Do not bury waste from meat-eating pets in food-growing areas or near water to prevent possible contamination.**

- **Do not add carnivorous pet waste to the compost pile. The pile will not get hot enough to kill parasites and other disease-causing organisms. It may also attract all sorts of vermin.**

- **Do not hose pet waste into the ground.**

- **Do not put out any type of pet waste for collection with yard debris.**

A good rule of thumb is to have one litter box per cat or no more than two cats sharing one litter box. Keep in mind, though, that if two cats share a box, it will need more frequent cleaning.

❶ **Cats like their privacy,** so it makes sense to put the litter box in an out-of-the-way place that minimizes odor and the tracking of litter.

❶ If you choose to flush cat feces, make sure only the feces goes down the toilet. Clay-based litter can clog up the toilet and your septic tank.

Take these steps to remove pet "accidents" from carpets:

1. Use a white towel to blot the damp area ASAP.

2. Apply a solution of ¼ teaspoon of dishwashing liquid and 1 cup of warm water with a white towel. Avoid over wetting.

3. Absorb moisture with paper towels, rinse with warm water, and repeat as long as there is a transfer to the towels.

4. Next, apply a solution of 1 cup white vinegar and 2 cups water with a white towel and blot dry. Stand on the towel to absorb moisture.

5. Secure a half-inch layer of paper towels on the area with a heavy object. When thoroughly wetted, replace. Continue to replace until towels no longer absorb moisture.

Try using an all-natural enzyme-based cleaning product as an alternative method. The **enzymes** actually digest the stain- and odor-causing proteins in the pet urine.

❶ Do not use ammonia or other cleaning chemicals with strong odors on the stained spot, as they do not effectively cover the odor and may encourage your pet to reinforce its urine scent mark.

❶ To **discourage a pet** from resoiling a previously soiled area, lay a sheet of foil on the spot for a week or two. It will be unappealing for your pet to step on.

☀ Save **hair-removal** time and effort by covering your pet's favorite furniture resting spots with a washable sheet, slipcover or bedspread. Remove and shake out pet bed blankets and pillows at least once a week. For easy care, choose bedding with a removable cover, or cover it with a machine-washable item.

☀ Use a rubber-bristled push broom or long-handled squeegee to push pet hair into rolls that can be picked up. A hand in a damp **rubber glove** rolled across the hair-covered surface is also effective. Also try stroking furniture with a damp sponge.

Make your own hair and lint remover with a wide strip of **sticky tape** wrapped around the palm of your hand, with the sticky side facing out. Press and pat down your furniture upholstery or curtains, using your palm. When that portion of the tape is filled with hair and lint, pull the tape around your hand so that you have a clean sticky spot. Repeat as necessary. This works great on clothing, too.

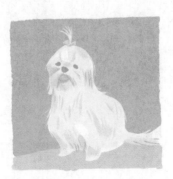

Pet-grooming wipes are great for cleaning DIRTY PAWS and wiping away the dander and excess hair that can cause human pet allergies.

Tips for Vacuuming Pet Hair

- Spray a static-removal product lightly over your carpet or furniture. Wait a few minutes, then vacuum as usual.

- If your pets have fleas, throw out or empty the vacuum bag outdoors after each vacuuming.

- Throw out or empty your vacuum bag when it is half-full, to prevent the vacuum from getting clogged with pet hair.

- If you are in the market for a new vacuum cleaner, ask other pet owners for recommendations. Be sure to look at cleaners that come with a turbo tool specifically designed to pick up animal hair.

pets, no pests

It's important that your rabbit, hamster, or other **furry friend** have a clean, dry cage. Look for a cage with a solid-surface floor and a large door or a lid that lifts off. Deluxe hard plastic structures with prefabricated tunnels and chambers may look appealing, but can be very difficult to clean.

Wash and refill water bowl or bottle daily. Clean up droppings with a wet paper towel; the dampness will keep dry droppings from turning into easily inhaled dust. Remove vegetables your pet has not eaten. Every other day, clean where your pet urinates. Remove dirty litter and replace.

Clean the whole rodent cage and everything in it weekly to prevent the growth of mold in the soiled shavings, which may make your pet sick. Completely empty the cage, and **wash and rinse** the bottom of the cage with mild detergent. Dry thoroughly before refilling the cage with fresh bedding.

☀ For easy cleanup, clip vegetables you feed to your pet to the wire frame of the cage.

☀ **Wear gloves** when cleaning up after your pet, and do not allow young children to clean cages.

Birds are not the neatest of pets, so it's important to establish an everyday cleaning routine:

- Use hot water and a scouring sponge to wipe food and feces off the cage, perch, and toys.

- Change the paper lining in the bottom of the cage.

- Wash the food and water bowls with hot, soapy water and rinse thoroughly. You may use a bird-safe disinfectant. Be sure that the food bowl is completely dry before adding seeds or pellets to prevent moldiness.

- Keep a handheld vacuum or a broom handy to clean up debris that has fallen from the cage to the floor. Minimize "fallout" with a cage apron or an office chair mat under the cage.

① Have a **second set** of clean, disinfected toys and accessories ready for immediate return to a clean, dry cage. Discard any items that do not come clean or need replacing.

① Line the cage with several layers of paper lining that can be removed daily, one at a time, as they get dirty.

Never use the self-clean feature of your oven around a bird; it can be deadly.

You do not need to remove the fish to accomplish the weekly aquarium cleaning. Take these simple steps:

1. Scrape algae off the inside of the glass walls with an algae scrubber or nonabrasive mitt. Also scrub rocks or decorations with algae. No need to remove them.

2. Trim excess growth and dead leaves on live plants.

3. Siphon off 15 to 20 percent of the water and replace it with clean tap water that's been allowed to sit in an aquarium-use-only bucket for 24 hours.

4. Use a gravel cleaner that vacuums up decaying organic matter.

5. Change the aquarium filter as recommended. Disconnect tubing and clean it with a filter brush.

If you find a dead fish, scoop it out immediately and bury or flush it. Remove all uneaten food within 10 minutes of feeding. Stir the gravel with your net to help particles in the gravel get into the filter. Position your **fish tank** away from windows, as sunlight can contribute to the growth of algae.

- Never use soap or other chemicals to clean anything that goes in your aquarium.

- Wearing household cleaning **gloves** will protect you against a bacterium that can be carried by fish and which causes open sores in humans.

pets, no pests

Understanding **pest behavior** and changing yours is the key to control. When tackling pest problems, always start with the least toxic method. Herbal solutions, such as peppermint or spearmint oils, can be used to repel insects. Nontoxic alternatives to pesticides also include a variety of traps and baits as well as ultrasonic technology, which uses high-frequency sound to drive rodents and insects away from your home without harming the human occupants.

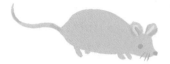

pets, no pests

Most insects and rodents prefer to live outdoors, but they will often seek food, water, and shelter in your home, especially in the colder months. Prevention is the best policy against household pests:

- Remove food and water sources and clean regularly.

- Make your home uncomfortable for pests.

- Employ tight-fitting doors, windows, and screens.

- Repair leaking roofs, chimneys, and pipes. Insects love moisture.

- Keep the perimeter of your home free of leaves, wood, mulch, compost, and heavy vegetation.

- Keep clutter to a minimum in garages, sheds, basements, and other storage areas.

Tracks and droppings are sure signs of a **rodent infestation.** You might also see gnawed cables or electric wires or damaged walls, floors, and doors. The sight of one mouse or rat is cause for action, because rodents reproduce rapidly; two mice can produce 2,500 heirs in just 6 months.

A mouse can pass through holes as small as a nickel; rats can squeeze into holes as small as a half-dollar. Try to determine how these rodents are getting into your home by sprinkling talcum powder on the floor in the suspect areas. Footprints or tail marks will indicate activity.

The following are general guidelines for handling mouse droppings:

- Do not sweep or vacuum mouse droppings; this can stir the dangerous hantavirus up into the air.

- Dampen the droppings with disinfectant and wipe them up with paper towels and a solution of water, detergent, and disinfectant. Double-bag the paper towels and seal before disposing.

- Wear rubber, latex, or vinyl gloves when you are cleaning up droppings. Before removing the gloves, wash your hands with disinfectant and then in soap and water; discard the gloves, and then wash your hands again with soap and water. If you are working in an area with poor ventilation, also wear a dust mask.

Poisons are not recommended for getting rid of rodents, for two important reasons:

1. The rodents often die and decay inside walls or under the house, resulting in a smell you really don't want to live with.

2. The poisons are hazardous to children and pets. Instead, deploy **mousetraps,** glueboards (very sticky glue on cardboard or in a plastic tray), or live traps. If you choose to use live traps, release the rodent at least 100 feet from your home, and make doubly sure it can't get back in by sealing it out.

You DON'T HAVE TO POISON your home with pesticides and insecticides to get rid of rodents and insects.

Indian meal moths, also known as **pantry moths,** enter the home through infested grains and other dried foods. Carefully inspect dried foods and packaging seams for webbing or larvae, which are sure signs of infestation. Discard infested food immediately and vacuum up any of it that may have spilled on your shelves. Use sticky traps designed to attract pantry moths.

❶ Place clothing infested with **clothes moths** outdoors in bright, hot sunlight. Or place items in polyethylene bags, squeeze out the excess air, and put the bags in the freezer for three days.

Clothes Moth Prevention

- **Keep closets and drawers clean.**

- **Store only laundered and dry-cleaned fabrics — perspiration and perfume attract moths.**

- **Vacuum carpets and furniture regularly, especially if you have pets, since pet hair is "good eating" for moth larvae.**

- **Avoid storing natural fabrics in areas with high humidity.**

- **When you're storing fabrics in sealed trunks, garment bags, boxes, or chests, store mothballs, cedar wood, or cedar chips with them. Replace or rejuvenate cedar with cedar oil every few months. Or store your fabrics with moth-repellent sachets made of dried lemon peels or dried lavender and cedar chips.**

Effective **ant control** begins with finding the ant colony's established trail to the food source in your house and following it back to the point of entry. Common points of entry include windows, doors, drains, and switch plates.

① A popular home remedy for deterring ants is **white vinegar.** Mix equal parts of white vinegar and water and carefully spray it around the ants' point of entry. Or sprinkle a line of cayenne pepper or cinnamon all around the point of entry; ants will not cross this line.

You can try tracing the **ant trail** back to the outdoor colony and spot-treating it with an insecticidal spray or dust. If you must use pesticides indoors, avoid sprays.

A safer approach is to bait ants and let them destroy themselves by taking the bait home to share with their fellow ants. Once you have determined the point of entry, just set delayed-action bait in the ants' line of travel. The ants will take the bait back to their nest, and eventually the nest will accumulate a toxic dose, which will eliminate the entire colony.

The simplest way to eliminate **spiders** is to disturb them often. Removing cobwebs makes adult spiders more vulnerable and removes egg sacs. Of course, not all spiders are web spinners; some are ground dwellers. Consider placing glue traps on either side of entrances where doors are opened frequently. General insecticide sprays are not effective.

MAKE YOUR OWN
Nontoxic Bug Spray

1. Mix 3 tablespoons of liquid peppermint castile soap with 16 ounces of water in a spray bottle. Spray directly on ants, spiders, and cockroaches to kill them.

As is the case for other insect pests, a good cleaning will go a long way toward preventing trouble with **cockroaches.** However, sanitation alone will not stop them. As disgusting as it sounds, roaches often "ride" into homes in grocery bags and food packaging. Even the cleanest homes can get them.

❶ The EPA recommends using **poison baits, boric acid, and traps** before resorting to pesticides. Place sticky traps under the refrigerator, dishwasher, and sink or in the places where the roaches run and hide when you turn on a light at night.

Following are a few ideas for getting rid of the cockroaches:

- **Simmer** catnip **in a small amount of water to make a tealike solution. Spray it around baseboards, on table legs, in cabinets, and under the lips of counters.**

- **Place a slice of bread in a coffee can with enough** beer **to thoroughly soak the bread. Lay the can on its side and leave it overnight in a popular cockroach "visiting" area. Empty the can in the morning and repeat as often as needed.**

- **If cockroaches are coming into your home through a drainpipe, pour a capful of** bleach **into the drain and close it up overnight.**

pets, no pests

The most effective method of **flea control** is a topical application. As fleas jump on your pets, they die. Vacuum frequently to get rid of eggs and larvae. If you do need to use a flea bomb or fogger, remove yourself and your pets from the house and be sure to wash water bowls and food dishes afterward.

MAKE YOUR OWN
Flea Spray

Score and slice a lemon, place it in a bowl, and pour 1 cup of boiling water over it. Allow the mixture to sit overnight, and then spray onto your pet.

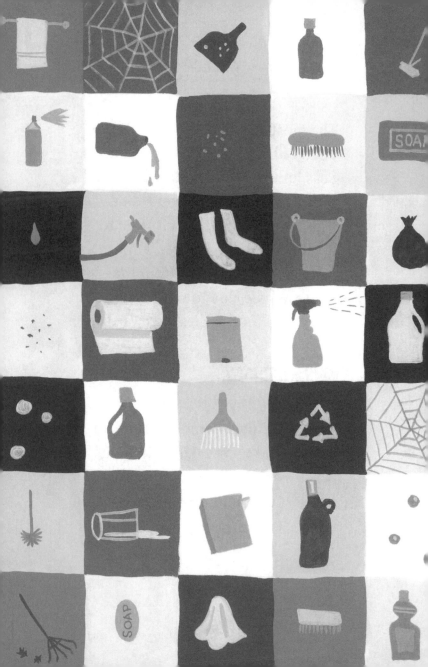

CHAPTER 7

Outdoor & Occasional

The exterior of your home, yard furnishings, and other outdoor property all need regular cleaning. Many outdoor cleanup tasks are "must-dos" on the spring and fall calendar. However, some cleaning and organizing efforts are only occasionally required, like those tasks that help dinner parties or holiday celebrations proceed smoothly. But seasonal celebrations needn't rattle the household. A little advance planning and organization can make the cleanup experience stress-free.

Give **your home's exterior** a good cleaning once a year. As a general plan, start with the roof (if it needs cleaning), and then move to the gutters, followed by the siding, the screens, the windows, and exterior doors and lighting.

If you live in a warm, humid mildew-loving climate or in a heavily forested area, you probably need to clean your roof annually. Otherwise, you run the risk of having the mildew destroy your asphalt shingles or cedar shakes. For safety reasons, most people opt to hire a **professional roof cleaner.**

When using a ladder, make sure it is STURDY and well secured. Never stand on the top two rungs.

Always clean your gutters out by hand, or you'll spray mud and leaves all over your siding:

1. Use a trowel to shovel debris out of the gutters into a garbage bag.

2. Next, flush the gutter in the direction of the drain, using a hose and sprayer attachment.

3. If the downspout is clogged, insert a hose into the lower end of the downspout and spray water upward. If that doesn't force out the clog, run the hose from the top of the downspout. If the clog still won't come loose, guide a plumber's auger or snake up the downspout and draw out the debris.

To remove dust and cobwebs from **siding,** use a garden hose with a sprayer attachment. To remove heavier grime, look for an all-purpose house wash in a container that attaches to your hose. Or use a long-handled scrub brush and a slightly sudsy solution of dishwashing liquid and water. Wash from the bottom up, and rinse from the top down.

If mildew is present on your wood siding, ask your paint dealer to recommend a house wash that includes a **mildewcide.** After washing, allow the house to dry for at least two to three days in dry weather before repainting.

If you take screens out in the fall, clean them before putting them into winter storage, and cover them to keep off the dust. Before reinstalling the screens, clean the windows and their frames:

- To clean screens that are only a bit dusty, simply spray the screens with a hose and sprayer attachment and air-dry.

- To clean very dirty screens, put a squirt or two of dishwashing liquid in a bucket of water. Dip a soft nylon brush into the solution and gently wash both sides of each screen. Spray them with a garden hose to rinse.

You can double the life of **patio and pool furniture** with proper maintenance. The easiest way to clean vinyl, plastic, and metal furniture is with a garden hose and sprayer attachment.

To clean **wicker furniture,** wet a cloth with a mixture of ½ cup of wood oil soap in 1 gallon of warm water and gently wipe one small section at a time. Use a toothbrush to clean between the weave. Rinse with a hose, turning the piece so that the water can run off. Wipe with a dry cloth, and allow 48 hours to dry.

Six Steps to a Clean Deck

A clean deck looks better and lasts longer. Leaves and debris that become trapped between the boards also trap moisture and make a deck susceptible to mildew or rot. Slippery green algae love a shaded deck, so keep that deck clean!

1. Clear the deck and cover any fragile plants growing nearby.

2. Sweep the deck free of large debris, and use a garden hose and sprayer attachment to rinse soil from the surface.

3. Wash the deck with a deck-cleaning product or a mixture of laundry detergent and water. Apply the cleaning solution to the deck and scrub with a push broom. Then rinse with the garden hose.

4. To remove algae (green) or mildew (black) buildup, mix a solution of one part bleach to four parts water and pour it over the deck, taking care not to get any of the bleach solution on nearby plants. Use a push broom to scrub off algae and mildew. Note that while liquid chlorine bleach will kill mold, mildew, and algae, it also can change the color of the wood. Concerned? Use oxygen bleach cleaner instead.

5. Rinse the decking thoroughly and allow it to dry for a few days.

6. Coat the deck with a penetrating preservative, such as a linseed-oil-based stain, which will be soaked up by the wood.

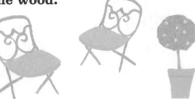

Pool Maintenance

A regular maintenance routine for your **swimming pool** will keep debris out of the water and regulate the balance of the chemicals:

- Run your pool pump 1 hour daily for every 10°F of the average day-time temperature; for example, on an 80°F (27°C) day, run the pump for 8 hours.

- Every day, remove debris from the skimmer basket and use a skimming net to remove floating debris. Clean the pump skimmer baskets once a week.

- All **filters** need to be cleaned once or twice a year. Follow your pool manufacturer's instructions.

- Brushing pool walls and floors helps prevent algae and bacteria from taking hold.

- Use a testing kit or strips to test chlorine and pH levels twice weekly. Adjust levels as needed.

- **Superchlorinating,** or shocking, your pool removes sunblock residue, perspiration, body oil, urine, and other contaminants. Shock your pool after rainstorms, after visits from a large number of bathers, and whenever the water looks cloudy.

- If algae forms, use algaecide products designed specifically for pools.

There's more to **cleaning your grill** than just scraping the grate with a brush or scraper.

Preheat the grill to high, and brush the grill with a brass-bristled brush. Then take a paper towel, fold it into a small, tight pad, dip it into a bowl of vegetable oil, and rub it across the bars of the hot grate, using a pair of long-handled tongs. Repeat as often as necessary, replacing the paper towel as needed. The grill grate should have a bright sheen of oil and the pad should come away clean when you're finished rubbing.

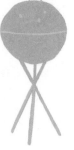

According to grillmaster Steven Raichlen, author of the award-winning *Barbecue Bible!,* the secret to SUCCESSFUL GRILLING is "Keep it hot. Keep it clean. Keep it lubricated."

Remove your **hammock** from its stand to clean. Lay it on a clean surface such as a picnic table. Use a soft-bristled brush and a sudsy mixture of dishwashing liquid and water to clean one side. Rinse well, and repeat on the other side.

① Before working in the garden or on your car or lawn mower, wash your hands and apply petroleum jelly liberally. The jelly will make it easier to wash grime off your hands afterward.

To remove leaves and debris from your driveways and sidewalks, start with a broom, rather than a hose, to conserve water.

To remove leaf or tire stains from **driveways and sidewalks,** wet the surface with a slightly sudsy mixture of dishwashing liquid and water and then brush the driveway or sidewalk with a push broom.

Oil stains on concrete and asphalt driveways can be difficult to remove. It's easier to remove fresh oil stains, so you should clean them up as soon as possible after you notice them.

To remove an oil stain, try one of these solutions:

- Blot up the oil with paper toweling. Sprinkle the stain with clay cat litter or cement mix, then leave it overnight. Sweep it up in the morning.

- Wet a stain thoroughly with a citrus-based all-purpose cleaner spray and cover it with several layers of paper toweling. Secure it with a brick or other heavy object, wait several hours, then rinse thoroughly.

- Use a paintbrush to apply paint thinner to older stains. Cover it with an absorbent material such as cat litter or cement mix. Leave it overnight and then sweep it up.

General Car-Washing Tips

- Remove dead bugs, bird droppings, and tree sap immediately.

- Use a special car-washing soap to avoid stripping the wax finish.

- Give your car a thorough rinse to remove surface dirt.

- To prevent streaking, wash your car in the shade and dry it with clean, soft towels.

- Wash and rinse one section at a time, starting at the top and working down.

- Wash and rinse cloths or sponges often in a bucket of clean water.

Some vehicle parts are more challenging to clean than others. Following are tips for the more difficult parts:

- Remove brake dust with a wheel-cleaning product designed for your type of wheels (for example, alloy or steel). Spray or brush on the product and then rinse it off in the time specified on the product label.

- Use a whitewall cleaner on tires. After washing, spray on a tire protectant.

- Shine chrome with a soft cloth dampened with distilled white vinegar. As needed, use a chrome polish.

- Dip a cloth in white vinegar and use it to clean road grime from windshield wipers.

Window **stickers and decals** can be very difficult to remove. Here are three tricks that work every time:

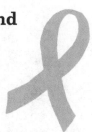

- Soak the sticker with white vinegar. Let it rest, then scrape off the sticker with a putty knife.

- Spray the sticker with WD-40, then wipe it off with a clean cloth.

- Spray the sticker with a commercial adhesive remover designed for cars, usually found at an auto parts store. Wipe it off with a clean cloth.

Birds are not likely to **SPLASH** around in a dirty birdbath.

A **clean birdbath** attracts more bird visitors and helps prevent algae growth, disease transmission, and breeding mosquitoes. For best results, clean the bath and change the water at least once a week:

1. Empty the bath completely.
2. Scrub with a small brush using a slightly sudsy solution of dishwashing liquid and water.
3. Rinse thoroughly to remove all detergent traces.
4. Refill the bath with fresh water.

1. Tossing **copper pennies** or a piece of copper pipe into a birdbath seems to help prevent algae from growing in it. It doesn't hurt to try.

It may be fine to run a **sleeping bag** through the rinse and spin cycles of your washing machine, on the gentle or delicate setting in cool water. If in doubt, however, wash your sleeping bag by hand in the bathtub with a non-detergent soap — pure soap, vegetable soap, or soap flakes — or a mild fabric wash for hand-washables. Then, let your bag air-dry. Warm, windy days provide the best drying conditions.

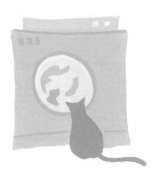

Vacuum tents **as needed to remove loose dirt. Spot clean with a sponge and warm water. If the entire tent needs to be cleaned, proceed as follows:**

1. Hose down the tent with clear water — or immerse it in a bathtub with cold water and a nondetergent soap or special tent cleanser.

2. Using a soft-bristled brush, scrub the tent gently.

3. Rinse the tent thoroughly several times to remove all soap residue.

4. Pitch the tent in the shade or hang it on a clothesline out of direct sunlight to dry completely.

5. Apply a coat of water repellent and let it dry completely before storing.

Whether you commute with pedal power or ride for pleasure, periodic cleaning of your bicycle will keep it at peak performance:

1. Use a garden hose to gently spray off any dirt and grime. Do not use a pressure washer, as this will blow out the grease that keeps your bicycle running smoothly.

2. Apply a cleaner/degreaser formulated for bikes to the frame, rims, drive train, and anywhere you have dirt or grime.

3. Rinse off the cleaner and dry the bicycle with a soft cloth.

4. Apply a bicycle-specific lubricant to your chain to prevent rust, shed dirt, and promote smoother and faster shifting.

It's hard enough to organize and shop for **holidays and special occasions,** let alone clean your home for overnight and party guests. But remember that the real reason for the season or event is to celebrate and enjoy. And the simplest way to avoid the pressure of preparing for holidays is to start early. Don't create unnecessary stress by leaving your cleaning to the last minute.

Some things, such as polishing silver and cleaning a guest room, can be done a month or more in advance. Dedicate one day each weekend for tackling preholiday cleaning jobs.

Involving your children in HOLIDAY cleanup will teach them to organize and tackle big jobs and may even evoke the SPIRIT of the season!

❶ Make a **checklist** of all the chores that need to be done in preparation for the upcoming occasion. In front of each chore, put an estimate of the time it will take to complete. If you have a spare hour, you can look for a task that you could accomplish in that time.

❶ Your home doesn't need to be **spotless.** If you are hosting an evening event, you can dim the lights to hide dust. Or, if you want to have an immaculate home but don't have the time to do it right, hire a professional cleaning service.

Make room for **holiday food** by cleaning out your refrigerator and pantry. Donate unneeded or unwanted pantry items to a local food bank.

☀ Pretend the holiday or special occasion starts one day earlier than it actually does. Plan to have everything finished by then. Then you can enjoy a day of rest before the festivities begin.

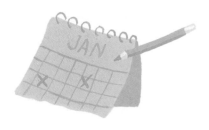

Company coming? If you have only a few hours to clean, make your kitchen and bathroom sparkle. Here are some quick cleanup tips:

- Clean toilets, sinks, mirrors, and bathroom floors and put out fresh hand towels.

- Close the shower curtain.

- Empty the kitchen and bathroom wastebaskets.

- Unclutter kitchen countertops and wipe them clean.

- Wash the kitchen floor.

- Go around the house with a laundry basket to collect any clutter. Stash the basket out-of-sight.

- Close doors to rooms that are off-limits to guests.

- Dim the lights for a twilight or evening party.

You can make the chore of cleaning up **after a party** easier by implementing a few strategies:

- Use good-quality disposable plates, utensils, glasses, and paper napkins.

- Place extra trash bags at the bottom of each trash container; when a bag is full, you'll have a new one at the ready.

- Keep receptacles handy for things like nutshells, shrimp tails, and toothpicks.

- If guests ask what they can do to help, assign the task of picking up trash, stacking dirty dishes, or wiping up the food-serving areas.

Because burning candles are so often part of household celebrations, "wax-ccidents" are inevitable. To remove candle wax:

- **From upholstery and carpeting.** Apply ice. Shatter the frozen wax with a blunt object and vacuum up the chips.

- **From tablecloths.** Freeze wax and scrape off with a credit card. Or place a paper bag over the wax and another under the fabric. Iron the top bag with a medium-hot iron until all the wax has been transferred to the bag.

- **From wood.** Place ice on the wax, scrape off what you can with a credit card, and remove residue with a cream furniture wax-moistened cloth.

Smoke odors are the most difficult ones to eliminate. The smoke particles are so small they penetrate everything. If you or your guests smoke in your home, you'll need to clean every surface to get rid of the odor.

To ventilate a smoky room, open windows and use fans. To help absorb lingering odor, place bowls of vinegar throughout the house. Leave them out overnight or longer, as needed.

Replace smoke alarm

BATTERIES at least

once a year.

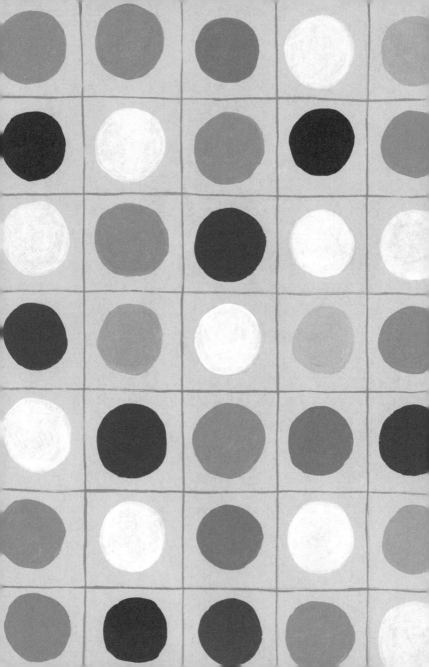

CHAPTER 8

Healthy Water & Air

Why should household cleaning stop with only what we can see? What about the air we breathe and the water we drink? We know a contaminated kitchen counter can adversely affect our health, but so can airborne allergens and impure water. Household systems require regular checkups to stay healthy. Knowing how to decrease pet dander, eliminate mold, unclog drains, and clean the systems that heat and cool our homes will not only reduce illness, but also save us money.

Studies have shown that the air in our homes can be even more polluted than the outdoor air in major cities. **Indoor air pollutants** can include tobacco smoke, vapors from household products and building materials, various biological pollutants — such as bacteria, fungi, molds, viruses, pet dander, and dust mites — and carbon monoxide and radon. Additional pollutants can be generated by everyday activities such as cooking with gas, dusting, and using spray disinfectants, cleaners, and repellents. These activities all add particulate matter to the air, which can create health problems for many individuals.

The air in your home should be continually exchanged with fresh air. This is tricky with newer, more energy-efficient homes, which not only keep out heat and cold, but also don't "breathe" like older homes that are not sealed as tightly. Ensuring **proper ventilation** is a good start in cleaning indoor air, particularly when you are using household cleaning products.

❶ If you can't open windows because of outdoor pollutants or traffic noise or because your air conditioner is running, use ceiling and **exhaust fans** to facilitate the exchange of fresh air.

Dog and cat allergens are found in almost every home in the United States, *whether or not* dogs or cats live there! In homes with dogs and cats, the levels of allergens are almost always high enough that they could trigger allergies or asthma. But even many homes without dogs or cats have dander levels high enough to provoke allergy symptoms. Where does this come from? Presumably it is tracked into the home on clothes and rubs off where people commonly sit. It also gets into the air. High-efficiency particulate air filtering **(HEPA) systems** in air purifiers and vacuums can help reduce exposure levels.

There are no cats that are hypoallergenic. Studies have shown, however, that light-haired cats cause FEWER ALLERGY SYMPTOMS than dark-haired cats — and that female cats produce fewer allergens than males.

Frequent cleaning can also help reduce allergens and irritants that cause **allergic reactions.** When you wipe countertops, for example, you are wiping away more than germs. You also wipe away pollen, pet dander, dust mites, and mold spores — the four most common indoor allergens.

❶ If you are the one who suffers from allergy symptoms, wearing a **face mask** during cleaning might help, as could cleaning a little bit at a time rather than everything all at once.

Dust mites live off human and animal dander and other household dust particles. They thrive in sofas, carpets, and bedding. Regular cleaning will minimize their population:

- Dust with a damp cloth and mop floors rather than sweeping.

- Regularly vacuum carpets, draperies, and upholstery with high-efficiency filters.

- Regularly deep-clean carpets.

- Cover furniture with slipcovers.

- Keep pets off the furniture.

- Choose washable curtains.

- Replace wall-to-wall carpets with smooth flooring and washable area rugs.

- Use a mattress cover and hypo-allergenic pillows.

Ways to minimize allergens in the bedroom include the following:

- Encase your mattress, box spring, and pillows in dust-mite-proof covers.

- Wash linens weekly in hot water (at least 130°F, or 54°C) to kill dust mites. Drying them on the regular or permanent-press cycle for 10 consecutive minutes also kills most dust mites.

- Put a hypoallergenic mattress pad on your bed, and wash it in hot water every week.

- Replace fuzzy wool blankets, feather- or wool-stuffed comforters, and feather pillows with synthetic or washable cotton blankets and antibacterial pillows.

- Wash pillows and blankets once a month.

Pollen is not just an outdoor problem — it also gets tracked indoors on clothing and hair. Saving outdoor activities for later in the day can help minimize exposure. Showering and washing your hair before going to bed will help reduce morning allergy. Because you keep the windows closed when in use, air conditioners reduce the entry of allergy-causing pollen.

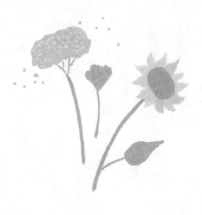

Mold can make it hard for your body to fight off infections, and can cause serious illness. So, cleaning up mold is a GOOD HEALTH investment.

Dank basements are the ideal breeding ground for **mold.** Mold generally appears as black or white stains or smudges. To find out whether a stain or smudge is mold, carefully dab at it with a drop of household liquid chlorine bleach. If the spot changes color or disappears, it's probably mold.

To clean mold areas larger than 10 square feet, or if the mold damage was caused by contaminated water, hire an experienced contractor. If you do the cleanup yourself, wear long rubber gloves, safety goggles, an N95 respirator (available at many hardware stores), and a shirt with long sleeves.

Following are some pointers for cleaning mold off different surfaces:

- Scrub furniture and other washable **hard surfaces** with hot, soapy water. Rinse with a wet rag, and dry thoroughly. Speed the drying with fans.

- To clean large areas of **concrete,** prepare a solution of ¾ cup of liquid chlorine bleach to 1 gallon of water. Open the windows for ventilation. Apply with a mop, and allow it to sit for 5 minutes. Then rinse and mop up the excess water. To remove small growths, spray the affected areas with straight vinegar and allow them to dry without rinsing.

- Take **rugs, upholstery, and mattresses** outdoors, brush off loose mold, and then vacuum. Afterward, wash the brush and dispose of the vacuum bag. Leave the items in the sun outdoors and air-dry. If mold is still noticeably present, make a very sudsy solution with water and soap, detergent, or carpet shampoo. Sponge suds onto the item, without getting it too wet. Wipe suds with a damp cloth and air-dry.

☀ You can sometimes salvage mold-covered clothing, pillows, blankets, or stuffed animals by laundering them in hot water.

Fending Off Mold

- **Clothing, paper, and furniture are the three biggest moisture magnets. Keep only what you need.**

- **Run a dehumidifier.**

- **In the summer months, open the basement windows.**

- **Avoid air-drying wet clothes in an already damp basement.**

- **Store firewood in a shed or garage, not in the house.**

- **Don't carpet the basement floor.**

☀ Absorb any musty odors left by previous mold outbreaks by placing a lump of dry charcoal in an open metal container, or set out a few small bowls of vinegar.

Carbon monoxide (CO) is a silent killer produced by burning fuel. Potential sources include room heaters, furnaces, fireplaces, gas ovens and ranges, and water heaters. Keep appliances in good working condition to avoid poisoning.

① **Carbon monoxide** has no smell, taste, or color, but you can do a quick check for signs of it. Look for rusting or water streaking on a vent or chimney, loose or disconnected vent or chimney connections, loose chimney masonry, a loose or missing panel on your furnace, inside window moisture, and debris falling from your chimney, fireplace, or an appliance.

Look for any problems that could indicate carbon monoxide release from **improper appliance operation,** such as a decrease in hot-water supply, your oil or gas furnace being unable to heat the house or running constantly, soot on appliances, or an unfamiliar or burning odor.

❶ The most important thing you can do to prevent carbon monoxide poisoning is to properly use and maintain fuel-burning appliances. A **carbon monoxide detector** should be used only as a backup.

The U.S. Environmental Protection Agency (EPA) estimates that INDOOR AIR POLLUTANT levels may be two to five times as high as the pollutant levels outdoors.

Many common household products contain solvents and chemicals that emit potentially harmful gases during use — and even during storage. For safety's sake:

- Avoid the use of aerosol products in your home.

- Do not use paint strippers and other strong chemicals indoors.

- Substitute nontoxic alternatives for cleaning and personal-care products.

- Use glues and other adhesives outdoors, or indoors only under very well-ventilated conditions.

- Do not store barbecue grills or their fuels in your living quarters or in an attached garage.

- Store solvents and pesticides outdoors.

healthy water & air

Portable air cleaners may be useful as a secondary means of removing home contaminants. Three general types are mechanical air cleaners, electronic air cleaners, and ion generators.

❶ When buying an **air cleaner,** look for the clean air delivery rate certification seal (CADR) on the packaging. It tells you how well the air cleaner reduces pollutants as well as the size of room it is suitable for. The higher the CADR number, the faster the unit filters air. You can then weigh the importance of other features to find an air cleaner that fits your needs.

We tend to take plumbing, heating, and air-conditioning systems for granted — until they don't work. The necessary cleaning routine:

- Vacuum grills and vents regularly.

- Change or clean filters monthly.

- Vacuum baseboard heater vents annually.

- Clean chimneys annually if you burn wood. Also check chimneys often for creosote buildup and clean when creosote is visible.

- Dust ceiling-fan blades monthly.

- Regularly vacuum portable gas and electric space heaters.

- Wash the filters of window-mounted air conditioners in warm water and detergent every two weeks; dry thoroughly before replacing. Regularly vacuum coils and clean drain pans.

A **clogged drain** is a dirty drain. If the clog is in a bathroom sink or tub — caused by hair, soap residue, toothpaste, or a combination of these materials — remove the strainer or stopper and any debris from around the drain opening. Using a flashlight, look down the drain to see whether a wad of hair is causing the obstruction. If so, reach in with a straightened coat hanger or a bottle brush and either push the hair down or pull it out. Then flush the drain with several gallons of scalding-hot water.

If you can't see the obstruction in a drain, try using a **plunger:**

1. Cover the drain opening with the head of the plunger.

2. To create a vacuum between plunger and drain, you need to "plug" other outlets. Stuff a rag into the overflow openings, stop up the second sink of a double sink, or clamp off the dishwasher drain hose.

3. Fill the basin with enough water to cover the plunger head.

4. Pump the handle of the plunger into the head several times and then quickly pull the plunger loose.

Repeat as necessary. When the clog clears, **flush the drain** with scalding-hot water to clear any remaining debris.

If the plunger method fails, try using a **hand auger.** The auger consists of a cable, which you feed down into the drain until it meets resistance, and a hand crank that lets you either push the obstruction down the drain or snag and retrieve the obstruction. Once the drain is clear, flush it thoroughly with scalding-hot water.

MAKE YOUR OWN
Drain Cleaner

Pour 1 pound of washing soda (find in the supermarket laundry aisle) in a bucket. Add 3 gallons of boiling water to dissolve it, and pour the mixture slowly, carefully, and directly into the drain.

The Sink Trap Fix

If you don't have an auger and the clog is in a sink, you can try removing and cleaning the sink trap — the S-shaped pipe under the sink — with a plumber's wrench:

1. Place a bucket underneath the trap, and then use the wrench to remove the trap pipe. Water and debris will drain into the bucket.

2. Use a bent wire to pull out any debris from the waste pipe.

3. Put the trap back together and flush the drain with hot water. This last important step not only rinses the drain and pipes but also refills the trap with water to prevent sewage gases from rising up through the drain.

Always try the LEAST TOXIC method for cleaning clogs first.

Someone's Got to Do It . . .

Don't use commercial drain cleaner on a toilet clog. Tackle a clogged toilet with a plunger:

1. If the toilet is overflowing, lift off the tank lid, pull up the float, and push down on the flapper at the tank bottom to stop the flush. Then turn off the water supply.

2. Bail out half the water in the toilet bowl.

3. Cover the drain opening with the plunger. Gently press the plunger handle down into the cup, release, and repeat until the water drains.

4. Pour water in the toilet to make sure the bowl empties.

5. Turn water back on, flush the toilet, and rinse the plunger in the flushing water.

If you can't clear the clog with a plunger, get out your toilet auger:

1. Place the auger in the toilet with the upturned tip going into the drain. Push down on the auger as you turn the crank clockwise.

2. Once you feel the auger pass through the trap, crank counter-clockwise to pull it back out.

3. Pour a bucket of water into the bowl to make sure it empties before you flush the toilet again.

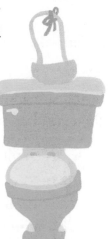

Kitchen drain clogs are most often caused by "plugs" of grease, embedded with food particles that obstruct the flow of water. To clear a grease clog, use a commercial drain opener with sodium hydroxide, which generates heat, to melt the grease and break it down so that it can be rinsed away.

For Safety's Sake

- If you do use a commercial drain cleaner on a kitchen clog, wear gloves and glasses.

- Never use a plunger or an auger during or after using a commercial drain cleaner, to avoid splashing the chemical on your skin, eyes, or clothing.

healthy water & air

While your **household drain system** carries water away, other household water systems deliver water where you want it and how you want it — hot, soft, or pure. Annual cleaning of the components of this system, including your water heater, water softener, water purifier, and drip-irrigation system, should be part of your **routine maintenance** program to ensure that you get the highest quality and maximum efficiency from them. If you are uncomfortable or unsure of what to do, hire a licensed plumber or specialist to do the work for you.

Flush your **water heater tank** annually to prevent the buildup of sediment and twice a year if you have hard water. Attach a garden hose to the drain valve and place the other end of the hose in a floor drain or on pavement outdoors. Carefully open the drain valve and allow the water to drain for 5 minutes. Then let the water fill a bucket.

If the water is clear and sediment-free once it has settled, close the drain valve and remove the garden hose. If you see sediment or discolored water, repeat flushing and the bucket test until the water is clear and free of sediment.

healthy water & air

❶ If you have not been flushing your tank on a regular basis, don't start now. The sudden flow of accumulated sediment can permanently damage your hot water heater!

If your **hot water heater** is rumbling or sizzling or the water it produces is rusty or black, there may be tank sedimentation or scale buildup on the elements. If you are a do-it-yourselfer, turn off the electrical power at the circuit breaker and turn off the water supply. Drain the tank and remove the access panel to the heating elements. Remove the heating elements, soak them in vinegar, and scrape off the scale.

❶ Keep all the operation and maintenance booklets for your household heating, air-conditioning, and plumbing systems in a **three-ring binder** and store the binder in an accessible place.

Create a log for recording the dates of cleaning, maintenance, and repair service for each of your household systems; tape the logs to each appliance, or store them in the household binder.

Now, you're prepared!

INDEX